The Other 23 Hours

The Other 23 Hours

Child-care work with emotionally disturbed children in a therapeutic milieu

Albert E. Trieschman
James K. Whittaker
Larry K. Brendtro

Foreword by David Wineman

Routledge
Taylor & Francis Group
LONDON AND NEW YORK

First published 2002 by Transaction Publishers

2 Park Square, Milton Park, Abingdon, Oxfordshire OX14 4RN
711 Third Avenue, New York, NY 10017

Routledge is an imprint of the Taylor & Francis Group, an informa business

First issued in hardback 2017

Library of Congress Catalog Number: 2001041596

Library of Congress Cataloging-in-Publication Data

Political Corruption : concepts and contexts / Arnold J. Heidenheimer and Michael Johnston, editors—3rd ed.
p. cm.
Includes bibliographical references.
ISBN 0-7658-0761-0 (pbk. : alk. paper)
1. Political corruption. I. Heidenheimer, Arnold J. II. Johnston, Michael, 1949-

JF1525.C66 P65 2001
364.1'323—dc21 2001041596

ISBN 13: 978-0-202-26086-0 (pbk)
ISBN 13: 978-1-138-53730-9 (hbk)

FOREWORD

Among other revolutionary developments of today's world is the so-called "knowledge explosion." So much is being written so fast about so many things that it is becoming well nigh irretrievable. Library scientists are facing the biggest headache in the history of their field in trying to solve the problem of information storage and accessibility. One consequently can never be sure that he knows what there is to know about many kinds of phenomena or types of problems existing in the modern world due to the chance that something exists in written form that simply cannot be found, so bulky is the load of literature.

How strange then to discover that in the field of child management, while one still cannot find much, the cause for this obscurity has shifted 180°. Instead of information retrieval breakdown because there is so much around, it is because there is so little. In the general torrential downpour of knowledge that drenches our libraries, there are only a few drops of information about how to live with children, "normal" as well as "disturbed"! Certainly it is not because the human personality has failed to perceive its fair share of being peeked at and probed out of the deep well of human curiosity. There are thousands of learned tracts about human functioning on hundreds of library shelves in most of the languages of the "developed" part of the world. Why, then, so little about "how to do," especially with children? Maybe because it is still more satisfying to describe phenomena than to try to influence how they work (unless money can be made, national pride exalted in some way, or war technology improved). Or maybe because there is not very much confidence, in spite of all the books in all the languages, about how much we know about human functioning anyway. Or maybe there are still undiscovered reasons that somebody is writing about right now, will publish, and will be hard to retrieve!

Whatever it is, or may be, that has resulted in this almost dry trickle of information and theory about how one may sensitively and intelligently guide the growth of children, the authors of *The Other 23 Hours* have decided to do something about it. They write in the tradition of the very few great contributors to the children's management field: August Aichhorn, Bruno Bettelheim, and Fritz Redl (from whom I was privileged to receive my own "boot training" in this field). That is, they are writing within the perspective of *the child and the life milieu:* how it is set up, what its critical ingredients are, how these impact upon the child, how the child copes with such impacts, and how these may be assessed and mediated so that the child's learning and growth are enhanced in the exchange.

This all sounds terribly specialized, sort of "hothousey," i.e., only to be conceived of in relation to very disturbed children living with very trained and dedicated staff. And, undeniably, the Walker Home is a place wherein the pathways of quite disturbed children who would stand little chance in the normal world of the average home, foster home, school, or camp and dedicated, trained adults do cross. But the "theory platform" that launches the living environment of *The Other 23 Hours,* those of us who work with it are convinced, is a *general* theory of how child growth and development can be supported and nourished by adults who *care* about and for children, not a special theory for disturbed children to be phased into their lives by highly trained and dedicated adults.

The common idea that only the sick child, and never the well, needs special emotional supports and helps from the adult is simply an error. For the well child is not immune from pile-ups of severe emotional intensity when overwhelmed by confusion and conflicts from *within.* Nor is he exempt from intensely complex reactions to experiences and events from *without.* Of course the child who is "sick," as compared to well, is more chronically bombarded from both these directions, within *and* without. But when the well child fails to meet such a "bombardment" adequately, he may look and behave much more like a *legitimately disturbed child than his usual normal self.* For instance, from *within,* the well child may experience a flare-up of an impulse to do or say something that he might not ordinarily consider acceptable. Or his mood may swing from depressed to elated, from apathetic and bored to "high" and overexcited. From *without,* consider the degree of regression that can be produced in perfectly normal children when they are confronted by a new sibling, lose a friend, experience the traumas of death or divorce. Or think of what a kid may go through at the hands of a bully or a group manipulator in the classroom, the betrayal of a trusted, admired friend, the torment of taking or not taking a dare, of peer ridicule, pre-examination panic, illness or injury—and a host of other highly probable external events that can never be anticipated as to exact time and place. Certainly, the normal kid can be expected to handle such crises either from within or without better than his sick peer *on the average,* but that does not mean *always;* and the critical issue for the well child is: *is he ready at the time they hit?* If not, he needs, quite unmistakeably, emotional first aid from the adult—parent, teacher, camp counselor (or what have you)—who is in charge of his life at that moment. The reader will find that what the authors describe in *The Other 23 Hours* as the everyday requirement diet, as far as child handling is concerned for their disturbed children, is transferable to the normal crises of normal childhood.

But crisis after all, whether from within or without, is the unexpected, the unplanned. This book is not only about how to meet unplanned events but perhaps, even more, about how to plan a day-to-day environment for children, albeit sick children. And here, again, the same old question: *only for the "sick?"* In a sense, and on a sliding and sometimes very slippery scale, every environment is planned where people live together. No environment really just falls together by chance. Every place where people live on a group basis, where there is some degree of interdependence, some mutual need confrontation and meeting, there has to be some *structure*. Otherwise there is chaos. This book is very concerned with structure and its effects on a day-to-day, even hour-to-hour basis, on the life of the child in the small group. Again, using the ego psychological orientation of Aichhorn, Bettelheim, and Redl (although these are not identical), the authors are concerned with demonstrating how the other 23 hours away from the one hour of clinical exchange that we call the psychiatric interview can be planned around the ego's function for the purpose of supporting and nourishing its functioning and development. Attentiveness to and implementation of very common structures in the "life web" of almost any child—routines, certain adult responses that the child may expect on a planned basis, certain activity programs—are here examined for what they both give to, as well as demand of, the ego of the child and how the balance between "giving to" and "demanding of" the ego of the disturbed child is arrived at. From here, the "transfer step" to the normal family setting, the foster home, the camp, and the classroom, all of which deal with many similar if some different structures—"markers" Dr. Trieschman calls them—affecting the lives of children, will be quite apparent to the reader.

Finally, a word about a most unusual event on the terrain of psychological theorization and its use that has occurred in the writing of this book, so subtly that it may escape the reader. Psychoanalytic ego psychology has for a long time recognized that creative thinking is long overdue on the implications of learning theory for the development and functioning of the ego. Not untypically the worry about the problem outstripped by far any intellectually and pragmatically responsible approaches to its solution. I use the term "responsible" advisedly. For what we have seen and is still occurring is a kind of holy war of the learning theorists against the psychoanalytic model *in toto* or even the tiniest exhalation of any of its constructs. And on the psychoanalytic side we have seen a panic-rage reaction against territorial invasion of the "clinical rights" to work with disturbed people. Both sides have displayed, ad nauseam, reams and reams of ad hominem argumentation in the place of anything that could even be mistaken for learned discussion. Such totalistic warfare is not only ridiculous but dangerous. In some clinical settings the wholesale application of totally untested operant conditioning techniques by workers who never saw a disturbed child before has rightfully horrified practitioners and in other pockets of the children's practice world psychoanalytic practitioners have only dived deeper into the bomb shelters of the reality-detached 50-minute interview. How refreshing then to witness the folksy, undramatic way in which the authors have injected their model with carefully controlled doses of both frames of reference, reflecting their basic allegiance all the way to *kids' needs* and not to the war of ideas and intellectual or professional narcissism.

The Other 23 Hours is a book that badly needed to be written. And read. Most urgently, it needs to be applied. For the field of child care in America, especially for thousands of Nobody's Children, away from home, is a sick shambles, a shabby, dried-up skeleton where is needed a *giant*, healthy and blooming and giving. This book is food for the mind of such a giant. Is it too much to hope that it may also help to make the American public want to build one?

DAVID WINEMAN

PREFACE

Nearly twenty years ago, when Fritz Redl and David Wineman were writing the preface to *Children Who Hate*, they stated their primary objective thus:

> Our main goal is to encourage the theoretician as well as the practitioner in all walks of life with children to take seriously the need to become more specific about ego control as well as about the techniques of handling child behavior . . . and we want to induce communities, children's institutions, and school systems to take new courage from an attempt to gain insights about children which have close bearing on the behavioral level and a practice in daily life.

This work along with its companion volume, *Controls from Within* (published together as a single volume, *The Aggressive Child*),[1] is today a unique and enduring classic in the children's field. The authors' work in Detroit and their subsequent publications about their early labors in residential treatment stand today as a pioneering effort from both a practical and a theoretical point of view. Not only were these two professionals intimately involved in the "life space" of the children at Pioneer House, their subsequent theoretical formulations dealt in great detail with the subtleties and perplexities of everyday behavior management with hyperaggressive children. It is sad to note that since the publication of

[1] Fritz Redl and David Wineman, *The Aggressive Child* (Glencoe, Ill.: Free Press, 1957), p. 15.

The Aggressive Child there has been precious little written about this most crucial subject.[2] It was our aim in writing *The Other 23 Hours* to bridge somewhat the gap that exists between the theoretical expertise of the professional clinician on the one hand and the very practical, often mundane problems of those who live with the children for the 23 hours apart from the therapy hour.

Many of our observations were made at the Walker Home for Children in Needham, Massachusetts. Walker is a residential center for severely disturbed, acting-out boys. The program includes individual psychotherapy, group therapy, and remedial education. It is also a training center for the mental health professions. The child-care worker bears the brunt of the therapeutic task in this setting and there are currently six full-time child-care workers on the staff. Another main source of our observations was the University of Michigan Fresh Air Camp—a treatment camp for emotionally disturbed and delinquent youngsters and a training center for students in the mental health professions—where two of the authors were associated for a number of years.

Essentially, the book attempts to do two things: to shed some light on the major routines of the day (wake-ups, mealtimes, and bedtimes) and to deal at length with two phenomena that are part and parcel of every children's institution: the temper tantrum and the therapeutic relationship. Additional chapters deal with the therapeutic use of games and activities with disturbed children, some pitfalls to be avoided by child-care staffs, and the rather involved process of observing and recording children's behavior. The initial chapter sets

[2] Some notable exceptions to this general lack of material are the numerous publications of Bruno Bettelheim at the Orthogenic School in Chicago. Probably the leading figure in residential treatment in America, his two most famous publications are: *Love Is Not Enough* (Glencoe, Ill.: Free Press, 1950) and *Truants from Life* (Glencoe, Ill.: Free Press, 1955); other significant contributions to the literature include: Gisela Konopka, *Group Work in the Institution* (New York: William Morrow, 1954); Henry Maier (Ed.), *Group Work as Part of Residential Treatment* (New York: National Association of Social Workers, 1965); Morris F. Mayer, "The Parental Figures in Residential Treatment" (*Social Service Review*, vol. 34, no. 3, 1960); and Susanne Schulze (Ed.), *Creative Group Living in a Children's Institution* (New York: Association Press, 1951).

forth the rationale for the therapeutic milieu and deals with its component parts and their application to the problems of the individual child.

In no sense do we intend *The Other 23 Hours* to present a definitive theoretical model to be followed studiously in every detail by other child-caring facilities. It is our firm belief that the institutional model that ultimately will survive is the one that remains eclectic and able to incorporate new theoretical formulations as they are developed. The theoretical underpinnings of this book derive essentially from three different areas: psychoanalytic ego psychology, the "life space" model of Redl, and some of the new sociobehavioral theories. If *The Other 23 Hours* is able to make a substantive and practical contribution to the statement that "the child-care worker is the most important figure to the child in the institution," then our major purpose will have been well served.

The authors of this book have all had direct experience as child-care workers in a therapeutic milieu. Our debt to the children we have worked with is most profound. The energy and anguish they bring to the tasks of being away from home and reordering their lives is impressive. It has been and continues to be a part of our education that is difficult to acknowledge adequately.

Our special thanks go to those clinicians and teachers who have extended our perspective beyond the fifty-minute hour —Robert White, William Perry, Samuel Waldfogel, Robert Young, Joseph Lord, Ralph Kolodny, Adrienne James, and David Wineman.

We are indebted to George H. and Irene L. Walker, whose philanthropy made Walker Home possible, and to the managing trustee, Richard G. Dorr, whose devotion to a life of service is quietly magnificent.

Walker Home would not exist as a residential treatment center if the staff of Parents' and Children's Services of the Children's Mission had not seen the need for such a service. Anne Cochintu, Shirley Bean, Marlene Lebow, and Ann Groves deserve special credit for closing the convalescent program and opening the treatment program at Walker.

The authors want to give special thanks to their families—the wives, Kathleen Whittaker and Nancy Trieschman, and young Thomas, Karl, and Matthew Trieschman—who lived with parts of this book and added realism to some of the notions in it.

Our greatest debt is to the child-care workers who have been our colleagues. Their skillful work with children has informed all of this book; their comments have contributed to each of the chapters. Nancy White, Marilyn Uleman, David Dorney, Richard Segal (who helped write Chapter VI), Michael Cranmer, Rosemary Merchant, and Winslow Myers were the first child-care workers at Walker Home. They were pioneers in both the excitement and difficulties of Walker's early days. Charlotte Ryan, Kathleen Whittaker, Margaret Komives (who helped write Chapter IV), Ruth Ann Smullin, and Barbara Riggs contributed to the ongoing process of assembling questions and answers about child-care work. Robert Bruzzese, John Magnani, and Dana Eddy are presently on the Walker Home staff and have made helpful comments on various chapters. All these people have been where the action is—at bedtime and mealtime and wake-ups. They have engaged disturbed children in activities and dealt with temper tantrums, and then they wrote notes on what happened! They helped "the other 23 hours" become a book; and more than that they helped those hours become a time of growth and change for disturbed children.

A special note of appreciation is owed Robert Paradise. First as a group work consultant and then as a staff member, he helped guide the development of Walker Home from the day we opened our doors to disturbed children. He helped write Chapter V and Chapter VI, and many of his thoughts have found their way into the rest of this book.

Many hands worked on typing the manuscript. Sib Lemack bore the brunt of this task with skill and perseverance. Peg Barnicle, Angela Akey, Mary Hayes, and Irene Brunke also worked on sections of the manuscript.

A. E. T.
J. K. W.
L. K. B.

CONTENTS

BIOGRAPHICAL NOTES

LARRY K. BRENDTRO, educator and psychologist, is president of Starr Commonwealth for Boys, residential treatment programs in Albion, Michigan, and Van Wert, Ohio.

ALBERT E. TRIESCHMAN is director of the Walker Home for Children, Needham, Massachusetts, and staff clinical psychologist, Children's Hospital Medical Center, Boston, and Lecturer, Clark University, Worcester.

JAMES K. WHITTAKER is instructor in social work, University of Minnesota, Minneapolis. He was formerly the assistant director of Walker Home for Children, Needham, Massachusetts.

DAVID WINEMAN is professor of social work, Wayne State University, Detroit.

I

Understanding the Nature of a Therapeutic Milieu

Albert E. Trieschman

> I should like to find out, not only what milieu is and how it operates, but also how we can describe it, how we influence it, and by what actions of all involved it is, in turn, created or molded. At the moment I am convinced of only one thing for sure—we all have quite a way to go to achieve either of these tasks (Redl, 1966, p. 94).

These problems face us nearly a decade after Redl posed them and more than four decades after professional work with children began citing the child's living situation as a therapeutic influence.

This chapter deals with these problems by presenting one kind of framework for understanding and utilizing a milieu as a therapeutic tool. Our notion is that the actions of adults with children and the adults' control of the environment can be coordinated to improve children's lives. Our framework is constructed for the adults who people a milieu: child-care workers, houseparents, counselors, nurses, social workers, group workers, psychologists, and psychiatrists. It is meant for all the adults who deal with children, or plan for children's living situations, whether they deal directly or supervise or advise those who do deal directly. Our major concern is the 23 hours outside the psychotherapy session—because that is when and where most of the milieu is.

Unfortunately we fall far short of complete answers to Redl's questions. Our look at the milieu is like a sea chart and some word pictures. It is unable to capture fully either the beauty or the turbulence of the milieu's many moods, and is hardly adequate to guarantee you will be a good sailor in that sea. If you grasp some of the excitement and power of milieu treatment and feel better equipped to participate in it, we will have succeeded.

The word *milieu* is our first hurdle. It is troublesome to pronounce and awkward to spell. What is it? Without being profound, let us settle on what we are talking about. We are describing a group living situation for children, specifically for children with emotional problems, children who must live away from home and whose lives are full of crises.[1] We are focusing on events that occur and processes that exist in such a setting. Moreover, we are thinking in terms of people using these events and processes as an effective tool to help children. It is our bias that much of what we say applies to child-rearing is general.

The chapter is divided into three sections. First, we deal briefly with the history of milieu treatment and the place of our notions of the milieu. Second, we consider the concept of the ego and its usefulness in conceptualizing the milieu's work of altering or changing behavior. Third, we consider some learning processes that go on between adults and children and some teaching forms through which adult actions and arrangements can occur in a milieu.

The Concept of Milieu

The daily events in a group-living situation may be viewed as foreground or background. The events and interactions of the day may be thought of merely as time-fillers between psychotherapy sessions, or only as providers of life necessities

[1] The ideas in this chapter are based mainly on observations and experience at the Walker Home in Needham, Massachusetts. The children we work with are usually diagnosed as acting-out character disorders, though some cases of severe neurotic acting-out and some with significant psychotic process have been served.

such as eating, sleeping, and recreation. *Or*—and this is our preference—the milieu can be thought of as the major impact that the institution has on the child. Whether as a time-filler or as a major therapeutic tool, a milieu exists in every group-living situation.

In recent years, every children's institution has claimed that they have a "therapeutic milieu," implying that they paid special attention to the therapeutic use of daily events. That claim is only possible since August Aichhorn's work in the 1920's. He first called attention to the planned use of the milieu as a therapeutic tool. Aichhorn (1955) wrote of the application of psychoanalytic ideas to the treatment of delinquents. Among many other things, he dealt with the organization of his training school, commented on grouping problems, and pointed out the significance of particular work assignments. He emphasized tailoring the environment to individual needs, as understood through psychoanalytic insights into individual children.

More recently the problem of milieu has been approached from a sociological viewpoint. The work of Stanton and Schwartz (1954), Erving Goffman (1961), and the Cummings (Cummings and Cummings, 1963), all with adults, has emphasized the importance of the social system that surrounds the patients. In between the vantage points of individual psychological and system sociological theory has come the classic descriptions that blend processes, events, and individual case episodes—provided by Redl and Wineman (1957) at Pioneer House, and Bettelheim and Sylvester (Bettelheim, 1949, 1955; Bettelheim and Sylvester, 1948, 1949) at the Orthogenic School. To all of these pioneers we are much indebted. They have taught us that the milieu can be a powerful therapeutic tool and have variously shown how individual psychological dynamics and the social system can be combined to manage and to change lives. Our contribution is dependent on their work.

We have not composed a new psychological or sociological theory. Rather, we have attempted to present a loose phenomenology of the milieu as a teaching tool. What goes on daily between children and adults is seen as an opportunity for therapeutic education or re-education of the child. The practitioners of the art of child care are our primary audience. They are the main teachers in a child-rearing milieu. Our assumption is that the rigidity, punitiveness, or over-permissiveness of some child-caring situations more often comes out of staff desperation than out of staff pathology or "meanness." Our hope is that better understanding of what is going on in the milieu, some sense of alternatives available to adults, and a means of communicating to fellow staff about what is going on will reduce that desperation. Hopefully, our ideas are stated broadly enough to keep the attention of readers from a variety of milieu situations: hospital wards, cottage systems, specialized schools, group homes and residential treatment centers.

Behavior and Ego Ideas

Children are placed in a therapeutic milieu so that we can help them change their behavior. We are using the term "behavior" in its broadest connotations and intend it to include intellectual and emotional aspects of childhood as well as actions or observable behavior. The changes we have in mind are not narrowly conceived as correction and even include growth and maturation. Without getting into the complications of diagnostic labels (mostly broad statements of what needs changing about the child), we can agree on some major categories of desirable change. We would like to help a child *stop* or diminish deviant, dangerous, age-inappropriate behavior. We would like to help him *start* or develop adaptive, productive, age-appropriate behavior. In short, we need to help the child to alter his behavior. The alternatives we teach are a complex and various pattern involving the interruption of deviance or "sickness" and the substitution of age-appropriate, productive, coping skills. Of course, this should not be thought of as a simple progression from bad to good, to better, to best behavior. A child's development should *not* be seen as a series of golden means in smooth ascendance to maturity: neat but not so neat as to be compulsive, has friends but can deal with solitude, asserts his rights but is not too aggressive, happy but can deal with sadness, etc. A series of twists and turns, ups and downs, extremes in one direction or another would be more appropriate descriptions. Add to that the complication that change for the better often leaves a child uncomfortable between old ways and not yet fully mastered new ways, and you can see all will not be smooth in this business of helping children change.

In what follows, we will explore the concept of alternative behavior, and consider some categories for identifying and communicating about behavior problems. Then we will seek guidelines for our teaching of alternatives from a developmental view of the child's ego and from a view of what daily events require of the ego. Finally, we will look for the areas of support to ego teaching that are available in the milieu.

We hope these sections will present both a means of satisfying children's needs and a means of helping children develop new competence to deal with life and learning. We are interested in curing mental illness, in serving children's needs, and in undoing the crippling effects of the past. But we are equally—perhaps more—interested in challenging children with the adventure of life, in promoting improved capacity to deal with the struggles of human existence, and in anticipating the opportunities of the future. The adults in a milieu are not just the suppliers of psychological medicine to empty, sick children; they are also the knowledged companions of children in an adventure full of challenges, obstacles, and opportunities. By combining giving something to and expecting something of children, we teach the lessons that promote love *and* competence.

The Concept of Alternative Behavior

For a moment let us concentrate on what we see, feel, and hear from a child and our need to change this behavior.

> Johnny came out to my car again today. As soon as I got out he pounded me in the middle of the back. He's been doing this a lot recently). It really hurts. I was puzzled because he always seems glad to see me.

Clearly, some alternative form of greeting is needed. But first we have to stop the pounding. To stop the pounding may be simply a matter of shouting at the child, refusing him friendliness, or actually punishing him. We hesitate to do those things because we value the growing positive relationship with the child. We could just tell him we don't like pounding, but that may prolong our martyrdom if he doesn't get the message. We should note here that stopping one piece of behavior and substituting nothing for it is a very difficult task for both the child-care worker and for the child. What could we substitute in the greeting situation?

This particular child-care worker told the child he did not like the pounding and decided on substituting handshaking, an act that he carefully practiced with Johnny. Johnny's need for physical contact in order to express his growing sense of trust was a hungry thing. The handshaking soon developed into counselor-child invented secret handshakes and later into elaborate hand-puppet games that were real affect dramas.

Without laboring the point, it is clear that stopping the pounding was facilitated by substituting another piece of behavior that provided similar satisfaction and was more acceptable, age-appropriate behavior. It is important to note that in developing this piece of alternative behavior, three activities were involved: *interruption* of behavior (don't pound me), *substitution* of behavior (handshaking), and *invention* of behavior (secret handshakes, hand puppet game).

Interruption of Behavior. Some behavior cannot be allowed to continue because it is dangerous to the child or adult involved, is disruptive to group living, or is destructive of the plant and equipment needed to help children. Adults will need to tell the child to stop such behavior and at times will have to stop the child. It is important both to stop some behavior for the child and to expect him to stop some behavior himself. This is obvious and need not keep us long. Basic honesty requires that you *not* offer an option to stop or continue (will you please, etc.) if you intend no option. Helping a child make choices is one significant teaching area, but not if you clutter it with phony choices.

Much behavior is not of the sort that clearly needs stopping. Some behavior is to be encouraged, other behavior just permitted, some ignored, and some prevented by the adult's control of circumstances.[2] We focus here on those all too frequent times when interruption is required, because they make our point clearly.[3] That is, that "control" of a child's behavior is a teaching opportunity; stopping something is an opportunity for behavior alteration.

Substitution of Behavior. The interruption of behavior often provides an opportunity for teaching a substitute piece of behavior. As with the handshaking, substitution refers to the teaching of some action (idea or feeling) the child already "knows" but does not use in the situation you are dealing with.

The choice of the substitute activity should be guided by some criteria—its fit with your best understanding of the child's intent, its social acceptability and age-appropriateness, and its capacity to diminish the alienation and self-defeat of the original behavior.

Skilled child-care workers get children to substitute mutual balance or leaning games for "hanging all over" adults. They may teach a child a way to ask to join a game instead of stealing the ball. They may bring a book or puzzle to an isolated child—in effect teaching, by substitution, some constructive uses of solitude.

Invention of Behavior. Invention refers to the teaching of alternative behavior that is not already a part of the child's repertory of actions (feeling, idea). Often it is the most advanced form of alternative behavior teaching. It usually involves a close adult-child relationship, with a considerable amount of identification of the child with the counselor. Iden-

[2] This is an indirect reference to the overall "control theory" of Redl and Wineman. See Redl, 1966.

[3] There are many different ways to stop or interrupt behavior. These techniques have been called "what to do until the ego comes" or "twenty things to try before hitting the child." See Redl and Wineman, 1957, "Controls from Within," and section III of this present chapter.

tification is meant to signify the child's copying of a competent model whom he admires.[4] In this situation the adult is sometimes able to design with the child a new piece of behavior. Substitution implies some "newness," in that an old piece of behavior is used in a new way. Invention involves "new" behavior to the child. The secret handshaking and the puppet play that Johnny and his counselor did were new activities to this boy.

Some teaching of alternative behavior by invention is involved in everyday occurrences such as playing a new game. The regulation and miniaturizing of aggressive play that occurs in board games like "Combat" is a case in point. Though some of the same basic instincts or impulses of the child may be involved in physical fighting and the board game, the invented behavior of the game is "new" in our sense of the word.[5] Teaching a child appropriate modesty instead of hiding at shower time, teaching a child sports expressions (like "kill the ball" or "smear the ball carrier") that are more socially acceptable angry noises, or encouraging a child to criticize a director so he will learn that he won't be destroyed for doing so—these are a few examples of "inventions" as a form of alternative behavior teaching.

There are many subtle versions of behavior inventions. One favorite "lesson" of a very skilled child-care worker was the teaching of "manners" and "cliched conversational forms." Some shy children avoid social interaction by "putting off" the other person (adult or child) with bizarre antics (grimaces, hiding, postures, etc.). After both adult and child recognized the intent of the behavior, this counselor would teach such children more usual and acceptable forms of I-don't-want-to-interact kind of interaction. "Hi, nice weather, see you around, fine, okay, nice to meet you, thank you, please, goodbye,

[4] Some of the complexities of relationship and identification are dealt with later in this chapter and in Chapter II.

[5] As with many useful ideas, the view that games can serve to teach alternative behavior has been independently developed by Eli Bower and his associates, to be used as classroom teaching tools for lower-class or disadvantaged children. They view games as a means of teaching ego skills to children and refer to games as mediating between primary process and secondary process thinking. See Allen, 1967.

you're welcome" can all serve to end or to avoid conversation, without needing to resort to scaring people off. In some respects it is the shy child who needs such forms and manners more than the bouncy, outgoing child who often charms people despite his acting out or aggressiveness. That such invented alternative behavior can lead to more basic changes—such as discovering it can be pleasant to interact with people—is incidental to our categories. At the least the child will know some useful behavior to alleviate his present shyness and will be prepared with behavior that will be useful if (when) he comes to desire more involvement with people.

The whole area of teaching a child how to cope with sadness is another possible subtlety. It is typical for disturbed children to be angry when it would be more appropriate to be sad. Helping a child gain competence to deal with loss—even in small matters such as "no mail today" or a broken toy—can be a considerable down payment on dealing with his life-depressing issues. When we model expressions of sadness, when we help a child seek replacements, when we help him to forget "that trouble" and go on to something else, we are inventing (sometimes substituting) alternative behavior that is an essential part of human equipment. It is interesting to note that we are now talking about helping a child to learn the behavioral skills to do what psychotherapists refer to as "the work of mourning" (Trieschman and Levine, 1968). And children separated from families have much mourning work to do. It is a truism that the "children who hate" often have many sad issues behind their anger.

Another version of inventing alternative behavior involves the use of books. Giving a child a book that provides fantasy material for an issue he is working on or a situation he frequently finds himself in can be a very helpful form of teaching. It may offer him socially acceptable indulgence of his situation—as when a very needy, nagging child is given a story to read about a king who has servants and slaves to do his bidding or stories about a child with many animal friends and helpers who do things for him. It may provide him with a sense of adventure and competence striving, despite his situation—as when a lonely child (perhaps even "rejected" by his parents) reads a story about an orphan who ventures into the world and triumphs over many obstacles. Many lists of children's books and stories, by age-level and issues covered, can be used by child-care workers to do this kind of behavior inventing.

One especially interesting use of this kind of alternative behavior involved the use of fairy stories (stories with knights, dragons, princesses, mean stepmothers, and kings) with a boy who was interminably in trouble playing male and female staff against one another. At the time he was doing this he was unable to talk about oedipal issues (family love triangles) with his therapist. In addition to being careful not to be exploited by this boy's "acting out," the child-care workers got the boy interested in adventuring fairy stories and folktales. Not only did his manipulation of the staff decrease with his growing interest in this reading, but he also began coming to his therapist with a great deal of issue-appropriate fantasy material. An additional benefit was that the staff felt—and were—involved in "therapy." Their teaching of alternative behavior was clearly a use of the milieu as a therapeutic teaching tool.

Many other examples of behavior interruption, substitution and invention will occur to adults working with children of different ages.

Teaching children to argue about sports or politics (he's the best second baseman in the league; my team is better than yours; all Republicans are against the poor; all Democrats are corrupt) is far more manageable than arguing with them about crucial institution rules or routines or having them differ with every adult direction. Banging fence palings is a more acceptable dribbling of hostility than gouging the cushions on the couch.

The fuzzy distinction between substitution and invention is not important. The name of the alternative behavior is not crucial. The notion that alternatives can be taught that help make adult-child interaction more livable and contribute to changing a child for the better *is* crucial.

If interruption, substitution, and invention appeal to you as ways to think about dealing with children's behavior, beware! They are not the whole story. Nothing that we have described so far works any profound changes in the children's psyches.

We have not changed angry boys into contented boys or shy ones into life-of-the-party types. We have made some situations more livable, and we have moved in the direction of healthier, more acceptable, age-appropriate behavior. Types of alternative behavior are only a means of describing one aspect of daily interactions with children. They are intended to indicate that, when faced with the problem of changing a child's behavior, you can think in terms of *teaching* alternative behavior. Though only a part explanation of a milieu, they begin us on our view of the milieu as a teaching tool.

We have not yet considered how we judged what to stop (e.g., the pounding was obvious) nor have we considered what to start (how substitutions and inventions might be selected). Moreover, we have said nothing of the means the adult might have of teaching alternative behavior. You did not know Johnny, the pounder, as an individual or as a member of a group in a particular setting. His poor sense of body control, his longing for physical contact, its connections to his early alcoholic parenting, and his recent but ambivalent willingness to experiment with trusting adults are all news to you. You did not even know how we identified and communicated about needing to teach some alternative behavior for the pounding. This kind of knowledge and communication of it obviously influenced the choice of interruption style and the choice of substitutions and inventions.

We should continue our notions about the milieu with some considerations of communicating about the behavior that needs changing.

Describing the Behavior That Needs Changing

If we are to be at all effective at teaching alternative behavior, we need descriptions of behavior that are closer to the child management arena than are the usual diagnostic statements. Character disorder, psychosis, hostile-aggressive tendencies, passivity, poor peer relations, etc. are useful statements when we are doing intake and when we are planning placement for a child. However, they do not indicate very clearly what our techniques or opportunities for teaching alternative behavior might be with that child. The addition of dynamic psychogenetics (e.g., "his primitive hostility springs from unresolved oral issues") is essential to our understanding of the meaning and intent of a child's behavior, but it too is unable to help in identifying specific opportunities for adults to intervene. What we need are child management oriented categories of information about behavior, more ways of organizing information about what the child is "like to live with," what kinds of "corrections" he "takes to," what his special sensitivities are, and what his tolerance for physical closeness or distance is. Redl (1968) has recently given us a rich set of categories for such information, and you are referred to this work.

In addition to "knowing the child" in these ways, it is essential that the specific opportunities and necessities for altering specific behavior are something we can focus on and communicate about. If the adults in a milieu are to be able to work together, they need to share information and pool skills around the management of specific pieces of behavior in their setting. A child-care worker can expound on the exasperation of trying to involve a passive, isolated child in the activities, and a psychotherapist can explain the roots of this child's passivity and isolation. But, unless we get into the specifics of the behavior to be altered, we may all be very "enlightened" while the child still sits in the corner. Similarly, teaching some alternative behavior to a child's "bad-mouthing" a particular counselor at particular times is a conceivable task. But dealing with "verbal or oral aggressiveness" is not something for which there is any general prescription.

The recurrent questions of what behavior to stop and what to permit or encourage are connected with what is "normal" and what is "pathological" for a child of a certain age, at a certain point in treatment, etc. Our categories of behavior description hedge this question by assuming that we already know we want to alter something and want to be sure we know what we are talking about so that we can start something better. The question of what to stop is dealt with, by implication, in our discussion of normal ego development and, directly, in Redl's (1966) and A. Freud's (1965) considerations of normality and pathology. Our descriptive categories are intended to cover "normal" naughtiness and pathology. There are plenty of occasions for stopping both and for needing to start some alternative behavior.

The categories of information we are about to propose are designed to aid in managing children. They cut across the various skill levels or specialties of the adults in a milieu. In dealing with specific behavior they help psychotherapist *and* child-care worker talk about specific opportunities and necessities for teaching alternative behavior. An example of their use is included in the chapter on bedtime routines (Chapter VI). Here we will just mention them.

1. *Locating the behavior in time.* If you are considering helping a child change his behavior, it is important to know the "when" of what you are discussing. Are you talking about behavior that occurs at bedtime—when during the bedtime routine?—in school, during board games, after failure, or maybe after success, at recess, or only on the playing field?

Perhaps it occurs only after or before a visit home, or only when a particular counselor first comes on duty. It might be a kind of behavior that occurs "when you first come to our place." Refinements in the time dimension are especially important when staff is talking about what to do about that behavior. It may seem to us as though "he is *always* doing that awful thing," but he probably is not. Strictly from the logician's standpoint, it is impossible to assign any refined notions of the cause or intent of behavior unless the timing of its occurrence and non-occurrence can be distinguished. We often cannot completely describe the "off and on" of behavior, and, of course, we then work on the basis of clinical hunches. We have to work that way quite enough as it is; let's not just do it out of our failure to pursue the information available to us in the pooled observations of the staff. *When* behavior appears is an important first step in planning management or in planning to teach alternative behavior.

2. *Locus among people.* At whom is the behavior directed—one particular other child, the group, only female counselors, adults, only male counselors? Who does the behavior involve? Maybe the behavior is always associated with a particular

pair or subgroup of children. Maybe it is "old kids" doing something to "new kids" or one particular child to everyone else because he wants to be old and new at the same time. All the knowledge we have about status and role systems in groups can help us come up with hypotheses useful in specifying a piece of behavior's locus among people. Another possibility is that the behavior is a solitary activity. Of course, this knowledge then helps us begin to specify *what* we might help that child learn in the way of alternatives. One knotty problem falls in this locus category—i.e., who started it? It is clearly important to try to answer this question, keeping in mind that the loudest or "naughtiest" youngster is not necessarily the initiator. Some other child's behavior may have "set him off." Both children may be able to profit from some behavior alternatives.

3. *Mode and pace of the behavior.* With the "when" and "who" aspect of behavior searched out, it is helpful to be sure that the adults involved in managing by planning alternatives know the mode of the behavior's expression. Sometimes we find ourselves talking about "aggression" without having specified whether we mean hitting, kicking, bad-mouthing, or throwing things. Certainly we should be clear about whether we are talking about verbal behavior, physical behavior, or both; and beyond that, we should specify parts of the body involved in this behavior and even what words were used. The planful teaching of behavior changes could hardly proceed smoothly if one person was talking about a "pounding with fists" and the other about a child softly muttering, "Go to hell."

The pace of behavior is another important descriptive dimension. We have in mind the intensity of the behavior—slow, aimless, quiet, preoccupied, even withdrawn *vs.* vigorous, intense, directed, even "driven" behavior. Dealing with behavior at very different energy levels requires different kinds of interventions. It is often necessary to gear the vigor of what we do to or with the child to the intensity of his behavior. We may want to help him learn alternative behavior that is up or down the intensity scale, but it is unlikely that we can teach an alternative at a radically different intensity level.

You probably could not get a child curled up on the edge of a game field to play at sports announcing the game, though you might be able to get a noisy heckler to participate this way. You probably can't get a "vilely" cursing child to speak his request in well-modulated, gentlemanly tones, but you might be able to get him to lower his voice and drop out the worst of the curses.

With just these three descriptive categories (time, people involved, and mode and pace), quite a bit of useful behavior alteration can be planned and accomplished. With children new to our setting or with new child-care workers, getting this information together may be about all that can be done. The next two categories require our "getting to know a child"—i.e., they require more than a single behavior incident to be used reasonably.

4. *Developmental level of the behavior.* This category involves clinical judgment about the *intent* of the behavior. What task of emotional development is the child working on? Is his behavior directed at answering the question can he trust an adult? Or is his intent more primitive and really an effort to define where his body ends and another person's body begins? Perhaps his behavior is an effort to "find his place" in the male-female dimension or about how he can relate to both mother and father figures (when he has different feelings and wishes toward them). Perhaps his efforts are multilayered and, in fact, directed at more than one emotional task. At this point we are stressing only that consideration of developmental level is important in dealing with behavior.

Unless we had known or guessed that one aspect of Johnny's behavior was his working on trusting adults, we might have missed an opportunity to teach him some useful alternative behavior; i.e., he would have failed to get through to us, and we might have acted in an antitherapeutic way. Realizing the "oedipal" developmental issue behind the behavior of the boy making trouble with the male and female staff, helped us select the "oedipal-type" reading material we gave him.

5. *Predominant mechanisms of defense.* What means of coping with a problem or an issue is the child employing? In this category we have in mind the various defense mechanisms and coping skills the child is employing in his struggle with the developmental issue. Avoidance, denial, reversal, reaction formation, magical thinking, repression, projection, intellectualization, etc.—this complex array of processes described in psychoanalytic theory is the major way of talking about "defenses" (A. Freud, 1946). It is important to note that these defense mechanisms are not pathological per se; in fact, they are the equipment of the ego and cope with problems. They are by no means simple, easily recognizable pieces of behavior—and we would deceive you if we implied this category was easy to use. It is linked quite closely with the developmental level category and takes some clinical experience to use. But the psychotherapist or consultant in your milieu will be in a much better position to make these developmental issue and defense judgments about behavior if both he and the staff share a set of descriptive categories of behavior. In turn, the clinical skill of a psychotherapist will be much more useful to a child-care worker if both professionals are clear about what behavior they mean. One especially helpful piece of information in this category is gained by noting the child's changing use of defenses. Such changes are often a good signal that the child is ready for alternatives—he may be trying out a new, more mature means of coping, or he may be under special stress and slipping back to more primitive defenses. Those times are among the best to teach alternative behavior, since the child is often "in the market" for some help with coping. Times of stress (whether from inner turmoil or outer circumstances) should be seen by the child-care worker as opportunities for teaching in the milieu.

The arrival of new children in the cottage or ward is quite instructive on this point. Similar to the phenomenon of "new baby in the house," the children in the milieu produce a lot of different-appearing behavior on the heels of the new arrival. On close inspection, it is often clear that their behavior is a mix of more mature developmental issues and defenses and some considerably less mature issues and defenses (regression). You find that Johnny variously seems more grown up (wants more independence and autonomy, explains very insightfully the new boys' problems, and how they are like his old problems, etc.) and more babyish ("devils" you for attention, needs your help constantly, goes back to old behavior like pounding you, etc.). It is often possible to capitalize on this mix by helping the child opt for the more mature alternative behavior.

The best use of our descriptive categories, of course, comes about when we are able to answer questions in all the categories. The interlocking of the information we gather as a staff begins to specify the time, pace, and mode, people involved, intent (developmental issue), and means (defenses) of the behavior we have to manage and the behavior for which we wish to teach alternatives.

Pounding a female counselor at arrival time by a boy identified with the aggressors of his past (defense mechanism of identification with the aggressor: the brutal parents), with the intent of working on the issue of trust (developmental issue)—that is, a behavior for which we can invent intelligent alternatives. Treating, "curing," or changing a boy's aggressiveness (unspecified) is a hopeless muddle.

What we have so far is some categories that help specify the intents of behavior and (by the connections to our "reconstructions" of history) the causes of behavior. That helps us plan to manage children through teaching of effective alternative behavior. A further consideration of developmental issues and defenses—in short, ego development—is our next task.

Guidelines for Ego-Based Teaching

We need guidelines in order to plan our teaching of alternative adaptive behavior to replace or supplement the behavior difficulties we have carefully described in our categories. We have chosen to guide milieu teaching by some notions of normal ego development, some notions of what tasks are presented to the child's ego by daily events, and some notions of where adults can look for support for "ego teaching." There are three sets of guidelines. One set is a view from inside a child's head; another set is an outside view; and the last set, a view from the standpoint of the child-care worker's concern for support of his teaching efforts.

Ego Development. We are not going to present a very full story of ego development. That would be a huge task and considerably beyond our needs here. Ours is a rather "folksy" summary of what is involved in ego development, with some indications of our particular point of view. It leans heavily on Sigmund Freud (1940), Erik Erikson (1950, 1959), Robert White (1963), Eli Bower (1966), and George Gardner (1966), but any distortions introduced by oversimplification (they do disagree on some points) cannot be blamed on their rich descriptions of the ego.

Freud dealt with three areas of mental functioning: the *id* (the inherited constitution, the instincts and impulses), the *superego* (prohibitions and inhibitions, originating with the parents, and considered a special part of the ego), and the *ego*. The ego is our concern. Its tasks, as assigned by psychoanalytic theory, are dealing with external events (through awareness, memory, learning, active modification of the external world, and avoiding excessive stimulation) and dealing with internal events (controlling impulses so that they are expressed when things are favorable in the external world). The impulses seek expression; the ego tries to provide satisfaction to the impulses. The origin of the Freudian ego is conceived as the result of the frustration of this satisfaction in reality. Much of psychoanalytic ego theory has concerned itself with the "defenses" that the ego uses against the impulses. Recently, Robert White has reviewed ego theory and added, to the ego, independent energies (not born of instinct frustration) which are promptings (like instincts) to explore and have effect on the environment. The child carries out this "effectance" behavior (unlike instincts) for its own sake and not because the activity reaches some particular bodily satisfaction and "goes away" until it is again aroused. Through this behavior, the child gains knowledge of the world, gets feelings that he can affect the world, and—over time—develops a sense of his competence to deal with things, people, and events. This energy, of course, does not replace the instincts. They still produce action, make effects, and bring satisfaction. Effectance behavior can work hand in hand with instincts. Its addition to the ego, however, allows us to conceptualize and explain some behavior and to do some teaching of behavior to children, without having to connect up with impulse satisfactions.

The growing ego then needs to develop an array of behavior (feelings, ideas) that can deal with the environment in such a way as to satisfy impulses *and* develop a sense of competence about dealing with people, things and events. Let us name large areas (via Erikson) of these necessary skills, because they are what we want children to learn.

1. A balance of capacity to trust and mistrust in favor of trusting, a sense of being able to get (from mother) and being able to give (satisfaction to mother)—*Oral Stage issues.*
2. A balance of autonomy over shame or doubt, a sense of bodily control and self-management—*Anal and Phallic Stage issues.* A capacity to affect his parents and be affected by them, language skills.
3. A balance of initiative over guilt, a sense of role in the family vis-à-vis mother and father figures—*Oedipal Stage issues.*
4. A balance of industry over inferiority, social learning (like sharing), precision learning skills (reading and arithmetic), capacity to work at something—*Latency Stage issues.*
5. A workable identity rather than a sense of self-diffusion —including sexual identity and social identity—*Genital Stage issues.*

These are a chronological series of "ballpark size" accomplishments going up into adolescence. Refinements occur when we consider specific ego tasks within these large areas. But in each "ballpark" there are issues of bodily satisfaction *and* issues of competence. For example, the baby in the Oral Stage needs to get nourishment to satisfy his hunger, but he also needs to sense that his crying and smiling have an effect on mother and to manipulate this effect competently. Of course, the solutions in each category effect the development of solutions in later categories. The reader should pursue the rich descriptions of the layered ego development of children, especially in Erikson and Gardner.

The children in residential treatment milieus have "defective egos." This means that specific tasks within these large categories have been poorly solved. As a result, we have the necessity, and the opportunity, to teach alternative behavior leading to better solutions. We look at the development of the ego as a structure of layered categories of problem solving abilities. Some of the youngsters we work with are still "hung up" working on the very early layers of ego development (the primitive children with considerable psychotic process); some of our children have proceeded through all the age-appropriate categories but have very few and rather weak specific task capacities in each category (poor ego strength, fragmented ego development) or a poor balance of solutions (some character disorders); some of the children in treatment milieus have many specific task capacities in each category, but the whole layered ego structure is quite a jerry-built, Rube Goldberg [6] piece of machinery, with many inefficiencies (many character disorders). We would like to think that, through teaching alternative behavior, we have a means of strengthening the ego's capacity to solve problems, a way of moving children along the developmental scale, and a technique for removing or replacing inefficient and unnecessary pieces of behavior in the "Rube Goldberg" ego. Our expectation is that some variation in ego strength, flexibility, and efficiency will exist into adulthood, especially in children who need to come into residential treatment. In short, we have no doubt that our treatment capacities are less than perfect. We expect that many of our children—like most human beings—will continue

[6] My colleagues have pointed out that everyone does not know Rube Goldberg cartoons. An example of them in words: A man in bed stirs, his toe pulls a string that opens a door which allows some food to roll down a chute, which gets a rabbit to move, whose stirring tips over a container of water, etc., etc., until a metal ball rolls against a gong and wakes the man. The point is many unnecessary steps to a desired result, a hundred places where something can go wrong. The board game, "Mousetrap," has contraptions that work thus.

to have their hang-ups and ways of falling on their faces. The teaching capacity of a milieu, however, can go a long way to increasing the child's knowledge of his problems and providing him with alternative, healthier solutions to them.

One important aspect of ego development that we should point out is the development of capacity to deal with feelings. The ability to cope with and use anger, frustration, sadness, longing, excitement, joy, and hope as meaningful parts of human equipment is often missing in our children. These tasks run through many stages and often require the most serious attention as we are planning alternative behavior.

In short, we like to think in terms of what "normal" ego development usually provides in the way of emotional task capacities; then we consider what the children in our setting are unable to do, do poorly, or do with great strain; and *then* we plan the teaching of some alternative behavior that will alleviate or eliminate their inabilities.

Ego Tasks Presented by Daily Events. In order to use the milieu as a teaching tool, it is important to speculate about what ego tasks the events, activities and occurrences in your setting present to children. What does a situation (especially a predictable recurrent one) demand of the child's ego? In later chapters we will examine some regular situations like bedtime (Chapter VI), mealtime (Chapter V), and waking-up (Chapter IV) partly from that standpoint. It is important to consider how much capacity to bear frustration a certain game involves (see Chapter III), and what certain aspects of your school schedule or specific subjects demand of a child's ego. Effective guidelines for child management and alternative behavior teaching demand that we examine our environment very carefully in terms of ego skills required to cope with it.

Sources of Support for Ego Teaching. These are exemplified in the chapter on bedtime (VI). Here we will mention them briefly. They refer to aspects of the milieu that child-care workers can call on in support of their teaching.

Relationships ("Shared Ego"). "Good relationships," much praised and demanded of adults working with children, are probably the most crucial aspect of the milieu (see Chapter II). The goodness of your relationship allows you to share or lend a child ego skills at various times. He may stop or start something because he likes you. Relationships, however, are not the only source of support for our teaching efforts. There are times when it is better to alter a child's behavior on some other basis than your relationship with him. His meager trust may make it more reasonable, in a particular situation, to ask him to do something because "we all do it that way" than to ask him on the basis of your "shared" relationship. There even may be times when a strong positive relationship should be "underplayed"; e.g., it would be foolish for a female counselor to overplay her positive relationship with a boy as a means of getting him to stop talking tough to the other guys; he may well have to be quite negative to her in order to "defend" himself from exposing his tender feelings at that point.

Group Mood and Structure ("Group Ego"). Knowledge of the structure of your group of children (tightly knit, clearly led, or multi-dimensional) and its mood (high, relaxed, antagonistic, cooperative) is essential to the child-care worker. A way of conceptualizing stages of group development is also important—i.e., newly formed groups "act" differently than long-established ones (Paradise, 1968). One support for ego teaching comes from sensible appeals to a child to alter his behavior on the basis of group functions when a group really exists (not just a gathering of individuals).

"Billy, please quiet down—we all want to hear the story." . . . "Everyone has to take a turn in the field if we are to play this game." . . . "Nobody else is doing that now." Such appeals are nonsensical when no real group exists or the child you are talking to is an outsider to that group. Of course, if the group mood is antagonistic, you are asking for trouble with such appeals. (See the further considerations of group mood and structure in Chapter VI and Chapter III.)

The Visible Culture of the Institution ("External Ego"). The culture, traditions, policies, and well-established rules and routines of your setting are another source of support for ego-based teaching of alternative behavior. It is possible for the child-care worker to call on these traditions in support of his altering a child's behavior.

At Walker Home we don't do things that way. At this place we always wash hands before eating or have a rest after lunch or tell a story around the campfire. It pays to be supporting yourself with real traditions, and not just universalizing what you want a child to do. You will quickly be exposed if you try. Of course, the establishment of a cohesive and visible-to-children culture takes time and hard work. When available, however, it is an important source of backing to the child-care worker's efforts to change children.

The Child's Own Ego Skills ("Ego Pieces"). This category of support refers to our careful descriptions of children's behavior. To the extent that we gear our teaching efforts to what the child presently is like in behavioral terms (his pieces of available ego functioning and their style) we are more likely to be helpful. The real source of support, of course, is our good sense and sound clinical judgment in matching behavior alternatives to the particular child that we are teaching.

Matching the vigorous handshaking that was based on an aggressive wish to try out trust in a relationship *to* Johnny's pounding promoted the learning of the handshaking. A whispered hello would have been a poor choice as an alternative behavior. Remember, Johnny had body control problems.

Before the phrases "shared ego," "group ego," "external ego" and "ego pieces" get us in trouble, let us be clear that they are intended only as a way to remember the sources of support to ego teaching, not as new kinds of ego structures. Up to now we have regularly referred to teaching and learning in our framework for a milieu. Now it is time we look at the processes involved in learning and the formats for teaching that are available for child-care workers to use.

Processes Involved in Learning and Formats for Teaching

In order for children to change, alternative behavior must replace or be added to old behavior. Acquisition of new behavior or change in behavior is one definition of learning. Psychologists have devoted many years of research and theorizing to learning. Here we will discuss learning from the perspective of adults interacting with children in a milieu. Our four *processes* of learning refer to ways one might describe the *functions* of these learning interactions. Our five *formats* of teaching refer to ways one might describe the *structure* of these learning interactions. The processes are a typology of how learning works; the formats are a typology of how the workings can be packaged.

Processes of Learning

The "what" and "when" of alternative behavior teaching are a good beginning, but now we need to consider *how* children learn. The following is a general description of the various processes that are involved in learning. It is not intended as a basic psychological theory but as a typology of the kinds of learning that go on between adults and children. Some readers will prefer to reduce our four processes to one learning theory (e.g., psychoanalytic theory or stimulus-response theory), and that is fine if you like such "neater" packages. Phenomenologically, however, these four classes of learning events do look and feel different to child-care workers. Although the adults and children involved may not always be able to choose which process they use, keeping them in mind does help adults vary their approach to children. They give us some options to consider when we are wondering if there is *any* way to get through to the child. In a difficult child-adult situation, rigid punitive tactics *or* total permissiveness can result from the sense that there is "nothing else to do." The following is intended to assure adults that there is more than one way to "get to" the child. We have called our four types of learning processes "Aha" learning, "Me-too" learning, "Stick-and-carrot" learning, and "Again-and-again" learning.

1. *Aha learning.* We intend this phrase to describe the va-

riety of learning experiences that are accompanied by the feeling of "Aha, I get it now." Insight is the term used to describe this process in psychotherapy. When a child (occasionally with a sense of suddenness) achieves a concept that has relevance to his feelings (past and present), we call it a *therapeutic insight.* Such concepts or ideas often have great significance because they may apply to "big hunks" of feeling and behavior and are useful over long periods of time. To be really useful, however, the idea must be visible to the child, not just to the adult. In other words, usually you must help it be visible to the child. What you "know" and the child doesn't is not an "insight" (except in your head). To the child it is only a diagnosis, your hunch, or even an insult to him (e.g., "You really hate your mother"). True therapeutic insight occurs mainly in the context of strong, long-standing relationship, with many life details available to both child and adult.

Recovering the memory of a particular event with his mother and how the child felt then and how these feelings are connected to his present behavior to a female counselor and doing this in some detail make up a therapeutic insight, no matter with whom it occurs (counselor or therapist). The "power" of such a generalization is obvious. It establishes a category of feelings and behavior that adult and child can use to restructure relationships, guide behavior, and understand the past.

Two things should be obvious by now: (1) Such insights are rather rare. If we are claiming that a child had three on one Saturday afternoon as he talked with you, you can be sure that we cannot mean "therapeutic insights." (2) Insights can occur in more partial form than our first example.

The child who takes note of how often he gets in fighting kind of trouble when he "fools around" with Bob in the early morning has achieved an insight of sorts.

Such *partial insight* is a more frequent occurrence than therapeutic insight. Our term should not be taken to imply that it is not important because it is partial. Achieving and using partial insights are more a part of daily experience than are the major restructurings of life we call therapeutic insights.

They can be one result of explanations by adults of a situation to a child. So far we have been implying that insights always have a significant emotional component; they usually do, but not always.

The child who discovers that it really helps to use a stick under a rock to move it (one kind of lever) has had an important kind of insight.

Such *cognitive insights* are connected with the feelings of efficacy and the sense of competence we mentioned earlier. Their component of emotion in the usual sense of anger, love, etc., is relatively small. In our dealings with children, there are many opportunities to provide experiences that promote cognitive insights. We can do this in our school programs and with the many mastery experiences of the activities in the milieu (on hikes, gardening, in the workshop), especially when we take the time to help the child "figure out" how the thing worked by his working it or thinking about it himself. (Don't rush to explain it all with your elementary physics.) Helping the child to achieve these cognitive insights by providing the necessary experiences and by helping the child verbalize his new knowledge is a significant process in teaching ego skills. It is a down payment on the child's future competence.

We do not mean to imply that insights are always pure examples of these three types. There are many mixtures and combinations; e.g., an intellectualizing youngster sometimes can use a cognitive insight as a partial insight into behavioral events.

Johnny and I (child worker) noted how similar his angry outbursts were to the way a dam works to generate power. (The teacher discussed dams in school today.) We had some fun with dam and damn that was right to the point.

At times, shifting conversation toward cognitive insight may be the learning process of choice. In an emotionally "hot" situation a useful point about behavior (including feelings) often can be made in an impersonal "cognitive" way that is less relationship endangering than even a partial insight.

Another useful time to remember the process of cognitive insight is in the discussion of prominent or national events with profound emotional impact (e.g., the assassination of a president). To pretend that we need not discuss such events overestimates the power of the milieu to monitor what children need to deal with, and our complete silence on the subject can have the effect of further alienating the children in our setting from a sense of participation in the world around them.

Explanations, through discussion of such events with children, can get hung up on the personal motivations of assassins. If we attempt to produce therapeutic or partial insights about these events, we sometimes get into personally damning (by implication) our angry impulsive children as "assassins." Cognitive insights (through sociological or political discussions) are often an excellent form of discretion. Along the way, we often correct some "wild" assimilations of world events into personal fantasies; e.g., a very "self-defeating" youngster in our setting was convinced that the United States president was sending guns to North Vietnam and United States troops to South Vietnam.

These three insight processes (therapeutic, partial, and cognitive) are processes that adults can think about using as they teach children about themselves (feelings and action) and the world. Partial insights, well communicated to children, are especially useful in explaining one group member to other children; e.g., "When Johnny comes back from a visit he is often kind of touchy and likes to be left alone."

Child-care workers can choose to use the insight process in working with children. They often do so when they opt to have exploratory conversations with children, when they seek with the child for an explanation of events in the milieu, and when they participate with the child in manipulating things to find out how they work.

We wish that it were possible to say that behavior can always be altered, and ego development served, with continual conversations, enlightening explanations, and "aha" experiences. Alas, it is not possible. Struggling to achieve fourteen insights of various types while keeping a six-man dodge-ball game from turning into mayhem and murder is about as hopeless a task as you will ever undertake. Fortunately, children do learn by other processes. Before we get into those, however, let us consider some of the advantages—and disadvantages—of insight as a process of learning.

The child-care worker's preference for working with insight processes is well founded. Achieved insights are very useful because they generalize well to new situations and because they avoid punitive engagement with the child. They also help the child sense his own participation in changing and learning. But there are disadvantages. Insights, especially of the therapeutic sort, are relatively rare. We are often in the situation of needing to alter behavior long before we have the kind of relationship and mutually accepted store of life details that allow true insight. Many times, the circumstances of the situation (many other children around, or it's time to go to sleep, or the child is 100 yards away) prohibit choosing insight as a process of teaching.

It is hard to imagine anyone shouting insights of any sort from the end of the playground to a child about to throw a rock at his playmate. But it is clear, we need to do something.

Even in the appropriate situation (e.g., adult and child conversation or calm group discussion), insight has some disadvantages. Therapeutic insights can be especially disquieting events. After a child unravels a knot of feelings and past events with an insight, he is often quite "raw" to any demands put on him or stress around him.

It can be very difficult for a child to participate calmly in a bedtime routine with other boys right after he has seen that his close and troublesome relationship with another boy is based on homosexual wishes.

Our point is not that insights are a poor process of learning to opt for but that they are only one process and must be used with care and good sense.

2. *Me-too learning.* Another important process of learning is the child's copying of adults. This can be more or less conscious or deliberate; it can be positive or negative (e.g., mak-

ing fun by mimicry); it can involve the copying of little bits and pieces of behavior or of large behavior sequences, including attitudes, opinions, and feelings; it can be a more passive or a more active process. What is clear is that children in our milieu do learn behavior by this means. The adults, in effect, propose many models of behavior for the children in their care. Although the adults can not control or determine which behavior the children will copy, they can exercise care and judgment in the models they propose. We should note that me-too learning is dependent on relationships, but not necessarily on only positive relationships. The defense mechanism of "identification with the aggressor," for example, is a term for copying the behavior of feared and hated people that you are dependent on. There are times when youngsters in our care are afraid of us and times when they "hate" us (e.g., when they are new in the setting or at particularly negative terms in their treatment). We should be reassured—and careful—that, even during those times, they are learning from us.

The temper-tantruming child may learn about reasonable expression of anger through the adults' model of firm angry tones in controlling him. There can be little doubt that reasonable expression of anger is an alternative behavior such a child badly needs to be taught. (See Chapter VII on temper tantrums.)

Perhaps it would be helpful to examine three different types of me-too learning in hopes that such discrimination will help adults be more observant of learning processes in the milieu.

Primitive Sameness. This kind of me-too is not a conscious copying of the adult, but rather an unconscious or unplanned assimilation of piece of behavior. It implies closeness between the adult and child and the dependency of the child on the adult, but does not necessarily include deep-level liking of the adult. (It can form a basis for liking, or positive relationship, later.) It does not assume an active intent to copy, and certainly no intention of mastery through copying a competent model. It is rather a passive process.

The "picking up" of phrases, words, little sayings that children do in the milieu is primitive sameness: "you bet," you better believe it," "up tight," etc. This process is really a very useful one in that children often pick up key expressions that either help us talk to them about a problem or, sometimes, actually function in their heads as a useful piece of behavior. An example of the latter is when a child learns our phrase and can use it with another child: "That is a two-man game and I don't want to play"—to a child who is tickling him.

Imitation. Here we have in mind conscious, planful copying of the adult's behavior. You won't always be able to distinguish it from primitive sameness, but it does deserve a separate description. We mean it to include both the copying of skills (using a hammer, throwing a baseball) and the taunting mimicry that children sometimes use with us. We have in mind both positive and negative imitation, but mean to restrict it to conscious behavior and to relatively small pieces of behavior. The process of imitation requires that the child see us as a separate person and "try on" the behavior he observes. Don't be distressed by the mimicry (unless it is part of an "uprising") because some of the behavior children "try on" in mimicry fits them and becomes a useful part of their wardrobe of coping skills.

Identification. We like to restrict this best of me-too learning processes to the copying of larger aspects of behavior (attitudes, ideas, "being a carpenter" instead of just using a hammer). It has both conscious or planful and unconscious or implicit aspects to it. It occurs usually in the context of a strong positive relationship.[7] It is a major means of influencing the lives of children in our milieu. Children copy aspects of our emotional and intellectual competence as a means of becoming more competent themselves. The adult's awareness of this process (especially separating it from the other more primitive "me-too" processes) is a powerful asset in using the milieu as a teaching tool. Our discriminating use of modeling behavior for children, within the context of a child identified

[7] By our descriptions, "identification with aggressor" would be a "primitive sameness with the aggressor." We have left out the terms "incorporation" and "introjection," though they do fit within our categories. The real point, however, is not terminological quibbles but our desire to make psychological theory useful to the child-care worker in the milieu.

with us, is perhaps the most efficient and powerful means of changing children for the better. It is much faster, once the identification is there, than the other learning processes and has no punitive overtones.

We could get a child to eat beans by achieving a cognitive insight about their protein value, or by rewarding their consumption and/or punishing him when they are left on the plate, or by putting him through bean-eating many hundred times; but the best and easiest way comes about when the child likes us, wants to copy us, and sees us eat beans.

We should add that insights, including therapeutic insights, often occur when a child is identified with an adult. Active competence-seeking (both emotional and intellectual) predominates in what we are calling identification.

Some identification processes occur in story-reading, and they should not be overlooked as a learning process. The heroes of adventures often become the mental companions of children in their struggles to become competent. This is especially true for children who are missing real people (like fathers) or for whom such figures are too "corrupted" by past experiences. The adults in the milieu often can mediate the relationship to such fictional heroes (by discussing the hero, finding books for the child, sharing an interest in the hero).

Using "me-too" learning requires careful observation of, and close participation with, children. It is especially important to make some effort to distinguish the various kind of "me-too's." When all that is available is "primitive sameness," one has to be careful not to expect a total degree of cooperativeness or mutual interest that is only true of identification. To do so may lead to disappointment on the part of the adult and, worse, to "blocking" the child from going on to more profound identification. However, our "me-too" distinctions should not be seen as mutually exclusive categories. Primitive sameness, imitation, and identification are continuing processes; one does not replace the other completely as a relationship grows, even though greater maturity is implied as one moves toward identification. All three continue to be part of human equipment.

3. *Stick-and-carrot learning.* This learning process involves planned use of rewards and punishments as a process by which children learn. We are not going to debate whether it is good or bad or if there is one special best punishment or many clever ways to "fit punishments to crimes." Issues of "bribery" or "punitiveness" will not be debated. We will not even consider the special effects of being sent to your room, being hit, or being "not guilty" (we "got" the wrong child). Redl (1966) has dealt with some of these issues quite fully. Our point here is that rewards and punishments for particular behavior in particular situations is a process by which some behavior can be changed and a process that will have to be used sometime. Using it is one of the options that adults have when they are considering how to teach a child something.

Any system of demerits or rules with consequences for breaking them employ reward and punishment as a learning process. Also, our disapproval of particular behavior has punishing effects and our approval has rewarding effects and usually alters behavior quickly, although not always in clearly predictable ways unless we consider many other variables (e.g., our relationship with the child, his view of whether we are rewarding or punishing *him* or the *act* he did).[8]

It is clear enough that we can choose this process as a means of changing behavior. Some of its advantages are the clarity of its message to the child (when we *are* specific and clear about what we are rewarding or punishing), its usefulness in situations when no other process is available or functioning in the adult-child relationship, and its capacity to build into the child some useful, nearly automatic control of behavior.

It would be "nice" if all behavior were guided by meaningful insights and other smoothly working ego functions but rather

[8] One might speculate that the success of "behavior therapy" in teaching new behavior to schizophrenic or autistic children is partly the result of the child's having no confusion about whether the punishment is for him (as a person) or his act. Such children often have very little sense of self as a person. It is hard, then, to imagine how behavior therapy alone could give such a child that sense of self without confounding its own technique.

"naïve" to confuse that wish with reality. "Superego functions" do exist and are not all bad, as popular psychology sometimes leads us to believe. Automatic prohibitions and inhibitions, though often implicated in neurotic functioning, are a natural part of mental equipment. They actually unburden the rest of the ego of some behavior control.

Our choosing to use reward and punishment should be guided by our knowledge that we may be building in an "automatic" prohibition or a rather stereotyped piece of behavior. Be sure it is a useful one to the child. The disadvantages of this reward and punishment process are real but have been oversold. It can, by exclusive use, promote automaton-like functioning in the child. Its overuse can result in much legalistic argument from the children as they try to negotiate our web of rules and punishments.

"Last Tuesday Bob broke my toy and you let him go outside and he didn't pay for my toy so I'm going out now." . . . "Billy hit Joey and only had to sit for five minutes, and don't think I'm going to sit here any half hour." Such "precedent citing" will eventually clutter up the whole milieu. Precious little useful behavior change (for the child) will result from your efforts to justify "justice."

To all the particular rewards you are familiar with (praise, candy, privileges, etc.) and all the particular punishments (restrictions to property, rooms, disapproval, condemnation, even lack of rewards), let us add some newer notions from experimental psychology ("Behavior Therapy," "Behavior Modification").[9] Do not assume that we have now become behavior modification experts or "reinforcement" clinicians. We just are not ruling out any learning process that might help us change a child for the better. On the other hand, we are not going to rewrite this chapter in reinforcement language and assimilate all our work with children into Stimulus Response or Conditioning terms. But we would like to suggest that the

[9] The work of Ferster and Simons has been especially interesting because it was carried out in a residential treatment center (Linwood Children's Center, Ellicott City, Md.). See Ferster, 1967, and Ferster and Simons, 1966. For another kind of reinforcement therapy, see Lovaas, Freitag, Gold, and Kassorla, 1965.

careful use of reward and punishment can be effective in altering children's behavior. The "behavior therapists" are careful (i.e., consistent and specific about the details of the behavior they are modifying in their differential use of rewards and punishments) and they have shown their willingness to have clinicians guide them in the selection of behavior to work on. They have used the concept of "natural reinforcers" for behavior that has intrinsic value to the child, recalling our attention to the capacity of competent completion of a useful act as a value in itself.

> You need not give most children candy for buttoning their own sweaters. They "reinforce" themselves with their sense of accomplishment.

Our point here is that in some teaching situations an adult may opt to try "behavior therapy" (consistent use of rewards, whether extrinsic like tokens, praise, or candy or intrinsic—natural reinforcers). It is also possible to reward an alternative behavior that is incompatible with the behavior you want to be rid of; e.g., the adult's approval of the handshaking with Johnny. Handshaking is behavior that is incompatible with pounding; you can't do both at the same time. It is likely that we already use versions of this learning process in some of our work with children, like rewarding all the isolated child's approaches to group fun. When we are careful about knowing the "lead up" to such behavior as tantrums, we sometimes can insist that the child use available alternative behavior. Punishing the use of the tantrum and rewarding the use of the better way can help us clearly communicate our expectation (hope) of his improvement to the child (see Chapter VII). Knowledge of behavior therapy principles may help us do it more carefully. Arguments about creating automatons of children apply to doing nothing but reinforcement therapy with children. They hardly apply to employing principles to guide our use of reward and punishment when we are already doing some of it in some fashion.

Several additional points on the subject of care in the use of reward and punishment: (1) Distinguish between rewarding and punishing; rewarding is preferable when possible and often it is by the considering an alternative incompatible behavior to reward instead of punishing the behavior you don't want. (2) Consider the implications of the particular rewards and punishments you use; e.g., you would not want some particular reward like food or money to symbolize all your approval or some particular punishment like isolation to symbolize all your disapproval. That would make it difficult for the child not to feel "unloved" when hungry and "punished" when alone. Hunger and solitude are human conditions which require mastery, not conditions of "moral turpitude." (3) Don't punish behavior unless you are willing and able to teach the child an alternative that you can help him substitute. (4) Be observant of the child's own use of reward and punishment. Some children come to treatment with elaborate internal self-reward and self-punishment systems that need careful taking apart (the jerry-built or Rube-Goldberg ego often has sin and repent systems that promote acting-out invitations to punishment). Make sure your use of reward and punishment doesn't confirm the system or add more useless "contraptions" to the child's functioning.

The use of reward-and-punishment learning *with care and thought* is a necessary part of running a milieu. It is really dangerous only when we have to pretend we never do "that kind of thing" and as a consequence hide its careless use behind a façade of guilty rationalization. One version of this façade is that reward and punishment are only for "control," and identification and insight are only for growth, love, and good relationships. Both halves of this proposition are near-sighted and destructive to a flexible and responsive milieu.

4. *Again-and-again learning.* The last of our types of learning does not have any pre-established labels, such as insight, identification, or reward and punishment. We are not even sure that it doesn't partake of many of the processes we have already discussed. What *is* clear is that some alternative behavior is learned as the result of a child being put through a sequence of actions again and again. In a milieu, and from the standpoint of adult-child interactions, such acquisition of behavior does need description as a type of learning.

Imagine that you are helping a child learn to swing on a swing It is unlikely that you do a great deal of insight-promoting explanations about the physics of a swing. You may demonstrate how you put your legs out at the beginning of a swing and how you tuck them back as you return (modeling behavior to promote imitation), but it is unlikely that you will rest your "lesson" on that process. It is very unlikely that you will rely very heavily on reward and punishment, though you probably do praise the correct move and say "no" to the wrong move. Most adults stand behind the child on the swing and sequentially and repetitively put the child's legs in the correct positions as they move the swing. We call that process of learning "Again and Again."

In a milieu there are many possibilities for putting children through sequences of behavior. Intentional, planful sequences are usually called routines. We think that when children are put through such sequences repetitively, they eventually learn to carry out the sequence themselves. It is important to keep that in mind when we plan routines. It would be foolish to teach children sequences of behavior that had no general usefulness outside our setting. Such behavior is really "institutionalism"—and avoidable. In planning sequences of behavior we are going to insist that children carry out, such as mealtime and bedtime routines, we should try to make them useful sequences. The behavior should aid the child's ego cope with the demands of the situation (see especially Chapter VI on bedtime routines).

There are also less visible sequences of behavior we sometimes put children in a milieu through. We might call them "implicit routines." We have in mind such possible sequences as the repetitive use of automatic punishments for a given behavior. To our horror, we sometimes discover a child has learned the sequence and now punishes himself (e.g., breaks a window and walks to his room). The overuse of insight-promoting conversation as an invariant consequence of misbehavior can also develop into children misbehaving and then announcing an "insight" ("I was upset. I talked about it. So there!"), and walking off.

Awareness of the again-and-again or "putting-through" kind of learning is valuable in planning routines and reflecting on possible rigidities in our environment. This kind of learning has a rote quality and it also has some similarity to trial and error learning (as children approximate the swing or exact routine). Of course, it is not a very rapid process of learning. As a process involved in well-planned ego-supportive routines, however, it can develop useful sequences of adaptive behavior. Our putting the child through the routine makes visible expectations for his behavior.

About Learning Processes in General. It is probably already clear that our kinds of learning often overlap and interrelate. For example, a child may achieve a very useful partial insight (e.g., he disapproves my act, not me) in the course of being punished by a person with whom he is identified. No one of these processes stands alone as the best way to help children learn. They are *not* a sequence of processes that culminate in only one mature adult way of learning (e.g., insight). All four kinds of learning remain a part of human functioning throughout life. Any milieu that used only one process (if that were possible) could hardly be helping children learn to be fully human. Such a milieu would leave itself open to exploitation by the children's need to maintain their symptoms. For example, if we rigidly sought "therapeutic insights" every time a child wouldn't do his arithmetic, you can be sure the child would learn to produce a worry, dream, or family problem every time you are ready to have him try arithmetic—and the worry would last for the whole lesson. Hopefully, an awareness of the various kinds of learning will help adults balance the milieu's use of learning processes. Understanding the various processes as they operate with individual children can be a great asset in promoting flexible intelligent engagement with children.

Formats for Teaching

Another way to look at what goes on in a milieu is to consider the ways we can package our teaching of alternative behavior. Interrupting, substituting, and inventing behavior can proceed by different teaching structures, as well as by different learning processes. The learning processes that are operating often are determined by the situation with that child; the formats or structures for our teaching are more often in the adult's control. What particular structure do we choose to use in order to "get to" the child? Do we promote behavior change by stating a rule, by establishing a routine, or by planning activities? Do we choose to talk it over with the child, or do we choose to deal with only surface behavior? Although these formats or structures obviously overlap and interrelate, it is helpful to keep in mind some "packaging" options that adults have in dealing with children.

1. *Rules.* Every group setting for children has some kind of rules. They range from elaborate demerit systems that rely on specific rewards and punishments to only a few necessary and "reasonable" rules for safety with no specified rewards or punishments. Our discussion is not an argument for one or another of these extremes of rule use. If we were to take a position in that argument, it would be that some situations in some settings with some kinds of children require adults to move toward one extreme or another, in order to operate effectively in the milieu. Here we only want to stress that rules are one teaching format by which we influence children, and to suggest several types of rules.

The considerations we have in mind are: who does the rule apply to (one child or the whole group) and how clear are the consequences for breaking the rule (automatic predetermined consequences *vs.* negotiated or indeterminate consequences). Combining these two variables, we get four kinds of rules that are useful structures for dealing with children in a milieu.

Group Rules with Automatic Consequences. These rules are the most usual kind and most settings have at least a few of them.

> Leaving property or the campus without permission means automatic restriction to campus and loss of allowance. Breaking a window means a fifty-cent fine.

It pays to be really specific about the behavior your rule applies to, and to make that specification clear to the children. There is no doubt that such rules hamper therapeutic involvement at times; it is equally true that they sometimes aid therapeutic involvement of the child.

The lonely child who briefly leaves campus in the company of a runaway is a case in point. We would rather commend or discuss his joining another person than punish his being off-campus. (However, it is possible that "doing a punishment together" builds some useful camaraderie.)

or

Consider the child who feels "hungover" with guilt after a misdeed. He may be better able to participate in programs after he has "shut down" his guilt through expiation of doing the punishment. Without it, he may feel a need to sin again in order to be punished.

Either of these viewpoints can be overplayed and lead to reckless justification of all rules or of no rules. Both viewpoints, tempered with clinical judgment, are important to keep in mind.

Individual Rules with Automatic Consequences. This kind of rule applies to only one child or, rather, to one particular behavior of one child. It is a rather infrequent use of rules, but at times may be the best ego "patch" we can make for a particular situation. The situation we have in mind is usually a fairly desperate one in which many other approaches have been tried.

We have in mind a child who has temporarily reduced most of his emotional life to anger and his expression of that anger to throwing rocks at people. Temporarily, we may want to specify this behavior to him and design an automatic consequence for engaging in it. It is important to be sure that we include an explanation of why it applies just to him and include a way for him to get off the rule. Enforcing the rule, of course, does not prevent our continuing to seek insights into the behavior or our working to promote alternative behavior.

We see this strict individual prohibition as plugging an ego leak with a superego patch. It is as if the child's psychodynamics and situation had temporarily conspired to prevent ego functioning about this particular behavior. For the sake of safe group living, we need to stop it and expediency dictates the choice of this packaging of reward and punishment. It is true another difficult behavior may soon begin to replace rock-throwing, but once we have the child altering his behavior, we are in a much better position to help him choose a safer alternative.

Individual Rules with Negotiated Consequences. Our directions to a child often include implied rewards or implied punishments, depending on the child's compliance to a rule. The child often asks us to specify what we will do if he does or doesn't follow the rule. Then the negotiation of the indeterminant consequences begin. Occasionally, this is a useful process, and we can help a child understand how rules work (an insight of sorts). More often, this negotiation is an ugly, angry conversation that would better be avoided. Children vary greatly in their "capacity" to do this kind of negotiation. Those who are "skillful" begin to sound like "con men"; those who are unskillful quickly become angrily desperate in their frustration over negotiation.

Group Rules with Negotiated Consequences. Though occasionally the adults may want to make a group rule and be free to deal out individually different consequences for infractions (having anticipated some exceptions or variances they want to make), this kind of rule making is very likely to promote a hodgepodge of legalistic argument from the group. It is the easiest kind of rule to make casually, but the most difficult to enforce. It often comes off as a veiled threat, and it produces much vindictive maneuvering by children and little opportunity for teaching alternative behavior.

In any group-living situation, adults will need to make and enforce some rules. The discriminating use of rules as a way to package teaching requires a careful assessment of children and group processes. The learning process involved in rules is usually reward and punishment. But the processes of insight or identification or "again and again" are not precluded by having some rules and using them consistently. Seeing that there is more than one kind of rule aids their discriminating use.

2. *Routines.* This package or format for teaching involves the

planning of sensible sequences of behavior that you help groups of children carry out around the regular events of the day (bedtime, mealtime). "Again-and-again" learning may predominate but the other processes we discussed also play a role in routines (imitation of other children, rewards, partial insights into trouble a child has). Other formats obviously are included in establishing routines (e.g., "rules" about when lights are out).

Occasionally, it is helpful to a child if you plan a special routine for him. He may have particular trouble with some time of the day—e.g., the transition from the school to the lunchroom—and establishing some routine for this time can sometimes "tide the ego over" the trouble spot.

We have dealt with routines in more detail in Chapters IV, V, and VI.

3. *Programming and Activities.* Chapter III deals with this "package" in some detail. Here we want only to point out that learning through play activities is perhaps the most natural format in which children acquire alternative behavior. The availability of a varied program of activities for groups and individuals is thus one of the most important aspects of the milieu. The ego skills mastered and the developmental tasks worked on in the activities are well worth staff effort.

Language of a favorite game can often be called on in management situations with a child—"You're on your last down now"—as a warning. Game substitutions for difficult behavior can often be taught; e.g., riddles and puns for a child who likes to "one-up" adults is better than his breaking rules. Leadership roles can be played out in some games. The insights gained and the identifications made on "the playing fields of Eton" probably explain those fields' claim to forming British men. Of course, board games and word games as well as athletics are included in the definition of activities.

4. *Managing Surface Behavior.* This format for teaching children refers to that magnificent range of life-space interventions described by Redl and Wineman (Redl, 1966; Redl and Wineman, 1957). The actions of adults in situations re-

quiring their intervention can range from "high signs" (shaking your head or making a stop motion with the hand), through distractions with humor, to actually "physically removing a child from a situation." We are suggesting that these life-space interventions can function as one form within which we teach children alternative behavior. Often Redl and Wineman's work is seen only as a means of adult survival with acting-out children, only as a means of keeping the situation livable. By contrast, we are proposing that when adults know a large variety of ways to manage surface behavior, they can begin to style their management to the ego needs of individual children and groups at different times.

5. *Conversations.* Talking with children is perhaps the most frequent way we package our efforts to help children. It obviously is a part of all the other formats we discussed. Here we will present three types of talking with children that are among the options available to adults in a milieu.

Psychotherapy Conversations. A lot more than talking goes on in psychotherapy (e.g., games, puppet play, finger-painting). However, our focus here is on the psychotherapy-like conversation. The pursuit of emotional issues in some depth and the consideration of the implicit connections between past and present are what we have in mind. Often these conversations are carried out by trained therapists or caseworkers (though occasionally child-care workers) in an office within the milieu. The necessity of making sensible connections between these conversations and what is going on in the milieu is crucial. Three significant milieu connections for psychotherapy are: (1) The amount of time the child has been in the setting (e.g., his acceptance of the placement, his peer relations in the setting); Brodie (1966) has presented a helpful set of stages for this aspect of gearing psychotherapy to the milieu. (2) The way the management techniques of the child-care workers with a child sometimes can confound progress because that particular technique happens to have powerful unconscious connections with the child's past experience; McDermott, Fraiberg, and Harrison (1968) have demonstrated this through a case presentation of a boy for whom physical holding reproduced the complex emotions of masochistic and homosexual beating scenes with his father. (3) Another consideration for psychotherapy in a milieu setting is dealing with the difficult behavior that occurs around times of change in a child's life. In the course of daily events, a child's return to his old symptoms (or the exacerbation of characteristic maladaptive behavior patterns) can be quite discouraging to adults in the milieu. They may treat this behavior-return with impatience and anger when, in reality, it often is a temporary effect of the child's discomfort with a new situation (e.g., a new adult or child in the milieu) or his discomfort with the first struggles with a new emotional task of development (e.g., trying to be a senior member of the group or trying to make relationships with children as well as with adults). At such times, the angry responses of adults can persuade the child to give up the struggle to master the new situation or emotional task. The psychotherapy conversation is an important teaching format to use at these times. It can help the child learn that, although he is having his "old troubles again," they are occurring around a new, worthwhile struggle. It also can help the adults in the milieu to deal with their discouragement. It may even help them to use alternative behavior teaching in the service of the child's new growing-up struggle rather than to see teaching alternatives only as a means of satisfying the child's old needs.

Life Space Interviews. Important conversations often occur outside of the therapist's office. Wineman (1959) has contributed a helpful description of this process, showing that it is useful both as an emotional "first-aid" technique and also as a format within which clarification and insight can occur. The exchange of information between office therapy and life space interviews is an important process. If different people are involved (therapist and child-care worker), as is usually the case, we must be careful that collaboration and cooperation are the watchwords, not competition to "penetrate" the child's psyche. Conversations (short or long) with children in the course of daily events are one of the key clinical skills required of adults in the milieu. Much of what we have already discussed could be repeated in describing how to guide conversations in the life space. The children in residential treatment often are "poor at" reflecting on themselves while sitting in an office so that, in fact, much crucial therapeutic engagement is left to occur in the life space. Ginott (1965) has recently written a great deal about talking to children, and some of this is useful guidance for life space conversations. Without belaboring the obvious, life space conversations are a teaching format that accompanies, aids, and assists almost all processes and forms we use to help children change.

One-Line Comments. In many settings, a few phrases or statements recur with considerable frequency. They become almost a part of the tradition and culture of the place. Often they begin as the "sayings" of an adult who is particularly effective in telegraphic-like communication to children. They are an undeniable asset in dealing with some situations with some children who know us well. As we mentioned under "primitive sameness," these phrases and sayings often become a useful part of the child's own verbal behavior. Some sayings that we have found useful are:

That's a two-man game. For two-child situations when your interruption may get cries of "you spoil fun," but situations in which you need to interrupt because the activity is about to explode or one child about to be exploited. Over time and with explanation, the phrase comes to mean that overt agreement and even rules are required for some activities.

Fair does not mean even. For the legalistic demands that a child makes when he insists on a replica of someone else's privilege. The phrase comes to signify an each-according-to-his-needs-and-abilities kind of fairness, not a legalistic duplication kind of fairness.

We care about you even when you don't. A handy rebuttal to the child who wants to end all engagement with you by saying, "I don't care, I don't care."

You're full of beans, or applesauce (or some favorite food). As a comment identifying a child's bouncy mood to him. This phrase becomes a pleasant way for you to make visible for the child, as well as yourself, his excitement level. It can help a child and an adult get together before trouble "spoils" things.

Last names vs. just first names. The varying "identities" of children who must live away from home is a real trouble to them. They belong to a family and to a group in your setting. In effect they are both Johnny "Smith" and Johnny "Walker Home." We have found it helpful to reserve using last names (with first names) mainly in addressing children at visiting time or other contacts with the family. It helps to set the stage for the child to anticipate and deal with his identity struggles.

I would like to trust you. As a conditional response to the child who is "baiting" the child-care worker with "You don't trust me" in order to get a likely-to-be-misused freedom or privilege. The phrase comes to signify a reasonable discussion of the basis of trust in a particular situation.

Our discussion of talking is far from complete. Talking with children, whether it is psychotherapy, life space interviewing, or a one-line comment, is obviously a key format through which alternative behavior can be taught and one which much experience and professional training goes into developing.

About Formats in General. One important aspect of a teaching format is who does the packaging. Children often have a different quality relationship with different adults in the milieu. Mayer (1960) has discussed this in terms of the various parent figures in the residential treatment center: "care parents" (child-care workers), "power parents" (director or board), the "middleman" (unit head, assistant to director), and the "transference parent" (therapist). Rules or conversations or surface-behavior handling obviously will have different impact, depending on which of these figures is involved. It is important that the milieu have a visible sensibleness to children, especially in regard to the way these various people are connected to each other and the children. Our focus in discussing formats has been the child-care worker.

The more intelligent options about child care that we can provide for adults, the greater the likelihood that children will be managed or changed with planfulness and flexibility. If adults have no rational options in their consciousness among which to choose, they can only operate with irrational unconscious processes. It seems quite unfair to provide child-care workers with only a few options about how children learn or about different ways to teach children and then criticize what they do as irrational unconscious processes ("he unconsciously provoked the child" or "that's his counter-transference"). Of course there are "good" irrational unconscious processes (our promptings to love) and "bad" ones (hate), and we are not proposing that it is possible to do without them; but it certainly seems "chancy" to leave the care of children mostly to the unconscious. An organized and flexible system of options with which to operate in a milieu gives the child-care worker some "ego skill" of his own to deal with children competently and lovingly.

Summary and Afterthoughts

We have presented a framework of notions about using a milieu therapeutically. Our argument runs as follows:

Children need adult help to change and grow and mature. In order to help the helping adults, we have suggested that the milieu be seen as a teaching tool. Stopping some behavior and starting other behavior were proposed as the key encounters of adults and children. Stopping and starting behavior was viewed in terms of teaching *alternative behavior*. Various types of alternatives—interruptions, substitutions, and inventions—were discussed. How to describe and communicate about behavior that needs changing was the next step. After developing some *management and teaching-oriented* behavior description, we connected altering behavior to the *concept of the ego*. We used this concept to view the developmental tasks of childhood and as a means of understanding how daily events present the child with ego tasks. The sources of support for ego-based teaching were then categorized (relationship, group mood and structure, tradition and culture, and the child's own ego pieces). And finally, we presented some descriptions of types of *learning processes* and types of *teaching formats* that exist in a milieu.

By now you will have noted that our ideas about using a milieu require a great deal of communication among staff. Time must be provided for such communication; i.e., regular staff meetings and regular conference time with child-care workers. And when this communication time is arranged for, the "right" things must be talked over. Dreary re-hashes of family history, old psychological test reports, and "he said–I said" therapy reports often do very little to guide our day-to-day work with children. Even their contribution to long-range planning is limited, unless meaningful connections with day-to-day events are made. Of course, periodic case conference reviews are needed, but they cannot be used as the only or main source of planning to change children's lives in a therapeutic milieu. They are not able to deal with the details of behavior changes nearly often enough or flexibly enough. They also may have the unfortunate side effect of limiting the participation (and sense of worthwhileness) of the staff who spend the most time with the children—the child-care workers. A great deal of the staff's communication time will have to be spent on the details of behavior management and behavior change. On what it all means, yes, but also on the processes and forms by which we can help teach alternative behavior, on thinking up alternatives that might help, and on considering our sources of support for this teaching. Pooling staff resources across professions, in order to consider alternative behavior, is time consuming. Our whole framework for the milieu is intended as a partial answer to the question of what to communicate about in order to use the milieu as a tool to change children for the better.

If we have sounded over-simplified or even a bit too directive in places, remember that this chapter is intended only as a framework of notions. That framework is built upon by the skill, knowledge, and enthusiasm child-care workers bring to the milieu. Do not mistake our framework for a summary of all there is to know about "milieu." Our ideas do not replace reading Redl and Bettelheim or any of those knowledgeable in milieu treatment. Important dimensions and enrichment have been contributed by many practitioners of the "milieu" art. If we have provided some notion of the sensible wholeness and potential teaching power of a milieu, we have succeeded. If you now feel that child-care work in the other 23 hours can really—but *really*—count towards changing disturbed and disturbing children into potential citizens, we are satisfied.

A postscript

You probably noticed that we have omitted many traditional areas of concern about milieu treatment. Among the most important omissions are: (1) Staff selection and organization. Who makes a good child-care worker or housemother, questions of the division of labor among staff positions, and questions of fitting together generic roles (the people who relate to children in many ways) and specialized roles (people who, for example only teach in classrooms or do office therapy). (2) The physical plant and equipment. Considerations of the importance of the physical structure, space, and things in helping children. (3) Work with families. Questions about the use of casework, family therapy, and conjoint therapy in conjunction with milieu treatment. (4) The community and aftercare. The details of carrying *outside* the institution and *after* the child's graduation from the milieu the gains he has made in the treatment.

We have various reasons for these omissions, but the basic reason is that our concern is mainly for the events and processes between adults and children in the daily living situation. Also, the answers to some of these questions vary considerably by the type of setting (a hospital ward or a cottage), by the professions employed (housemother, nurse, or child-care worker), and by the age and diagnosis of the child (preschool children *vs.* adolescent; psychotic *vs.* character disorder). Our *certainty* is that there is more than one good, coherent way to answer each of these questions, depending on what setting, which children, what kind of families, and what professionals you have in mind. Our *hope* is that our notions are basic enough to apply helpfully to many kinds of milieu.

References

AICHHORN, AUGUST. 1955. *Wayward youth.* New York: Meridian Books.

ALLEN, LAYMAN. 1967. Rules and freedom: games as a mechanism for ego development in children and adolescents. Report of Workshop F, 44th annual meeting of the American Orthopsychiatric Association. Obtainable from the author, 1407 Brooklyn St., Ann Arbor, Mich.

BETTELHEIM, BRUNO. 1949. A psychiatric school. *Quarterly Journal of Child Behavior,* 1(1): 86–95.

———. 1955. *Truants from life.* Glencoe, Ill.: Free Press.

———, and Emmy Sylvester. 1948. A therapeutic milieu. *American Journal of Orthopsychiatry,* 18(2): 191–206.

———, ———. 1949. Milieu therapy indications and illustrations. *Psychoanalytic Review,* 36(1): 54–68.

BOWER, ELI. 1966. The achievement of competency. In *Learning and mental health in the school.* Washington, D.C.: Yearbook of the Association for Supervision and Curriculum Development of the National Education Association.

BRODIE, RICHARD D. 1966. Some aspects of psychotherapy in a residential treatment center. *American Journal of Orthopsychiatry,* 36(4:) 712–719.

CUMMINGS, JOHN, and ELAINE CUMMINGS. 1963. *Ego and milieu.* New York: Atherton Press.

ERIKSON, ERIK. 1950. *Childhood and society.* New York: W. W. Norton.

———. 1959. Identity and the life cycle. *Psychological Issues,* 1(1): 1–171.

FERSTER, C. B. 1967. Transition from animal laboratory to clinic. *Psychological Record,* 17(2): 145–150.

———, and JEANNE SIMONS. 1966. Behavior therapy with children. *Psychological Record,* 16(1): 65–71.

FREUD, ANNA. 1946. *The ego and the mechanisms of defense.* New York: International Universities Press.

———. 1965. *Normality and pathology in children.* New York: International Universities Press.

Freud, Sigmund. 1949. *An outline of psychoanalysis.* New York: W. W. Norton.

Gardner, George. 1966. The behavioral disabilities in adolescence. In Sylvano Arieta (Ed.), *Handbook of psychiatry.* New York: Basic Books.

Ginott, Haim G. 1965. *Between parent and child.* New York: Macmillan.

Goffman, Erving. 1961. *Asylums.* Chicago: Aldine Publishing Company.

Lovaas, I., G. Freitag, V. Gold, and I. Kassorla. 1965. Experimental studies in childhood schizophrenia. *Journal of Experimental Child Psychology,* 2(1): 67–84.

McDermott, John F., Selma Fraiberg, and Saul Harrison. 1968. Residential treatment of children: the utilization of transference behavior. *Journal of the American Academy of Child Psychiatry,* 7(2): 169–192.

Mayer, Morris Fritz. 1960. The parental figures in residential treatment. *Social Service Review,* 34(3): 273–285.

Paradise, Robert J. 1968. The factor of timing in the addition of new members to established groups. *Child Welfare,* 47(9): 524–529.

Redl, Fritz. 1966. *When we deal with children.* New York: Free Press.

———. 1968. Are we barking up the wrong data tree? Twenty clusters of action-relevant observations as basis for decision-making in behavioral crisis situations. Paper presented at the 45th annual meeting of the American Orthopsychiatric Association, Chicago, March, 1968.

———. 1964. How do we know this is normal? Unpublished.

———, and David Wineman. 1957. *The aggressive child.* Glencoe, Ill.: Free Press.

Stanton, Alfred, and Morris Schwartz. 1954. *The mental hospital.* New York: Basic Books.

Trieschman, Albert E., and Bernard Levine. 1968. Teaching the competence to deal with loss. Unpublished.

White, Robert. 1963. Ego and reality in psychoanalytic theory. *Psychological Issues,* 3(3): 1–210.

Wineman, David. 1959. The life space interview. *Social Work,* 4(1): 3–17.

II
ESTABLISHING RELATIONSHIP BEACHHEADS

Larry K. Brendtro

Although it is widely proclaimed that "relationship" is central to therapeutic work with disturbed and delinquent children, this term is certainly not well understood. Some would argue that the word is so vague and diffuse as to be devoid of any real significance. Others, who feel that their clinical experience attests to the existence and importance of "relationship," would still maintain that it is unnecessary or even undesirable to try to specify something so personal and intuitive as relationship. Yet, anyone who has had the opportunity to observe new child-care workers attempting to "establish relationships" would certainly agree that many of them do not seem to know what it is they are supposed to do or how they might go about it. If "relationships" are indeed important, then it seems important that we understand what it is that we are talking about and how the child-care worker "builds relationships." We shall open our discussion by considering the problem behavior that disturbed children typically bring to the worker-child interaction. We shall then define what we think is meant by "relationship" and how it influences children's behavior. Finally, the major portion of the chapter will attempt to provide the child-care worker with some specific ideas as about how to establish and use therapeutic "relationships."

The Concept of Relationship

The Relationship-Resistant Child

With many of the children we encounter in residential treatment settings, we find ourselves hampered by a circular problem: we are told that our major tool is the "relationship" we offer, yet these youngsters' major difficulty is in the development of appropriate relationships with adults. Such children seemingly cannot or will not allow the establishment of the "relationship" that seems essential for therapeutic change. In our attempts to interact with these children, we are confronted with communication barriers, their unresponsiveness to social reinforcement, and their rejection of the adult model.

Barriers to communication. These youngsters are often secretive, guarded, seclusive, aloof, withdrawn, or deceptive. They act as if they cannot trust, understand, or be understood by the adult. They often erect a deceptive front or maintain a barrier between themselves and the adult, effectively keeping the adult at a distance and interaction at a minimum. This pattern is examplified in the following account by a child-care counselor attempting to communicate with a new boy in a therapeutic camp:

> I approached Jim on his first afternoon at camp to try to involve him to the programmed activity. He had been sulking around the cabin, refusing to talk with anyone or to answer questions, even staying away from meals. Although others had tried to communicate with him to no avail, I initiated an extended monologue about his interests (which I knew included drag racing), the camp, his reasons for silence, and anything else I could think of. He only pulled his pillow over his head to shut me out. When I persisted, he got up, walked out, and left me talking to the empty cabin. We left him alone, and he came to supper, yet maintained an uninvolved, predominantly mute stance for the next few days.

Unresponsiveness to social reinforcers. Many of these youths seemingly could care less about obtaining the adult's approval or disapproval. They appear immune to the usual social rewards of praise, attention, and smiles, as well as the usual social punishments of disapproval, scoldings, and frowns. If they do respond to rewards and punishments, it is only to the more concrete varieties, such as money or food. Such a child is described in the following example:

Since there was quite a bit of trouble on the trip to Lincoln Park, Millie wanted to talk to the boys about this upon their return. "I am disappointed in the way some of you boys acted on our trip," she told them, and most of the fellows looked guilty. Not so Mark, who paid not the slightest heed even though he had been, as usual, the main troublemaker. Likewise, in situations where she would praise Mark for some acceptable behavior, he would either completely ignore her praise or sometimes even begin to misbehave again.

Rejection of the adult model. Such children do not readily identify with the adult's behavior or ideals, but rather tend to exaggerate their differences from the adult, often by behavior opposite to that of the adult. They reject the adult model of socially desirable behavior, even more neutral adult behavior, such as style of dress or language. While there are normal developmental differences in the degree to which children imitate the behavior models provided by significant adults (e.g., normal adolescents are less likely than younger children to model adult behavior), still these youngsters seem not the least bit inclined to use the adult as a behavior model.

In his novel about teaching in a deprived, inner-city school, Hunter writes of a teacher's attempt to influence his adolescent boys in their attitude about good music. He brought his own personal collection of records to school and played them to the boys. Not only did they fail to identify with Mr. Edward's musical interests, but they went so far as to destroy all of his prized collection:

"Smash the friggin' thing!" someone shouted.

"No, don't! Stop it, stop it! You don't know what you're . . ."

The record hit the wall, splashed off in a dozen flying black pieces. Someone else was at the record case now, and Edwards was rushing across the room trying to stop him. . . .

[Long after it was over and they were gone] the tears kept

coming because the records were a part of Josh Edwards . . . (Hunter, 1954, pp. 171–173).

Not all disturbed children display such extreme difficulties in interpersonal relationships. In fact, many are as easy for the average worker to interact with as would be a group of normal children. But a large number of children encountered by the child-care worker present these difficult problems, and the worker will need something more than friendliness and good intentions in order to work effectively with them.

What Is "Relationship"?

Almost everybody agrees that "relationship" is important, yet there is little consensus on what this term means. Since in this chapter we shall consider how one goes about "establishing relationships" with maladjusted children, it seems mandatory that we attempt to clarify what we mean by this global term. Continuing from the foregoing discussion of the "relationship-resistant child," we suggest that it is profitable to consider "establishing a relationship" as consisting of three elements.[1]

1. Increasing the child's communication with the adult.
2. Increasing the child's responsiveness to social reinforcement provided by the adult.
3. Increasing the tendency of the child to model the behavior of adults.

Thus, when a worker speaks of having "established a relationship" with a particular youngster, the implication is that this adult (a "significant other" in contrast to adults in general) communicates readily with the child, is a strong social reinforcer to the child, and is a behavior model whom the child imitates. When the worker speaks of "not having a relationship" with another youngster, the implication would be that one or more of these three elements is lacking.

[1] While one might argue correctly that a relationship is a two-way phenomenon, our discussion will concentrate upon the effect which the relationship has upon the child rather than on the adult. This is not to minimize the importance of the adult's role in the relationship, particularly that which has often been referred to as the "counter-transference."

Each of these elements of a relationship is considered separately in the discussion below.

Communication. The first element of a "relationship" is communication between two individuals. To the extent that communication is neither impeded nor distorted, then the necessary foundation of a "relationship" has been established. Communication is not only verbal (talking, corresponding) but nonverbal (gesturing, physical contact). The existence of communication can be observed in numerous ways (e.g., the child may constantly seek out the adult, talk to him, wave to him, greet him, ask questions, jump on him, etc.). To the extent that the two parties in the relationship have engaged in a large amount of communication, a number of private symbols often develop—symbols not generally understood by outsiders (e.g., nicknames, special meanings for certain words or signals, private jokes, or even a private language).

Social Reinforcement. A second element of a "relationship" is the increased susceptibility of one person (i.e., the child) to the other person (adult) as a source of social reinforcement. The child-care worker who "has a relationship" with a certain child possesses certain reinforcing properties which are not possessed by non-significant others (such as strangers). In this situation, the child generally strives to obtain the approval and to avoid the disapproval of the adult. Even when no concrete reward or punishment will be forthcoming. The previous experience of a child with adults is perhaps the main determinant of the amount of influence social approval or disapproval will have upon his behavior.

Modeling. A third element of a "relationship" is the greater tendency for the child to imitate or model certain behavior patterns of the specific adult. This modeling is something more than an attempt to gain the adult's approval, since it may occur in situations where the model is not present (e.g., a child may continue to model his father's behavior even after the father is dead). The modeling frequently occurs without the awareness by the child (e.g., a child adopts his father's facial expressions or style of walking) and also without any intention of the adult to teach the child the behavior. For example, research suggests that parents who discipline their children's aggressive behavior by physically punishing the child may actually be providing a model for more physically aggressive behavior by the child.

It should be clear from the foregoing that the existence of a "relationship" places the child in a vulnerable position; he can readily be influenced for better or for worse. Thus, it is not enough for the worker to establish a "relationship" with a child, but he must also see to it that he uses the "relationship" in a therapeutic manner. While a hostile child-care worker (a) may communicate a great deal with a particular youngster, (b) may be a potent social reinforcer to the child, and (c) may provide a model to the child, yet the net impact upon the child can easily be negative.[2] Therefore, even if we know that a "relationship" exists, we know nothing of the impact the "relationship" might have upon a child.

How Does "Relationship" Influence Behavior?

In our opening chapter we discussed four learning processes which the child-care worker can utilize to influence the behavior of children. These were the processes of insight learning, reward and punishment learning, identification-imitation learning, and "putting through" learning. Depending, of course, upon the child and the situation, it was our premise that the child-care worker must be attuned to any or all of these four learning processes.

A crucial task of the child-care worker is to help the child learn new ways of behaving; therefore, a prime aim in "establishing a relationship" is to facilitate this learning. Why is "relationship" so important in our work with these children? Perhaps because it allows the adult to more effectively utilize three of the processes of learning.[3]

[2] Such relationships have been described in psychoanalytic writings as "identification with the aggressor."

[3] In the opening chapter we discussed a fourth process of learning, which was labeled as "again-and-again learning." This process of learning does not appear to be as dependent upon relationship as are the other three processes of learning.

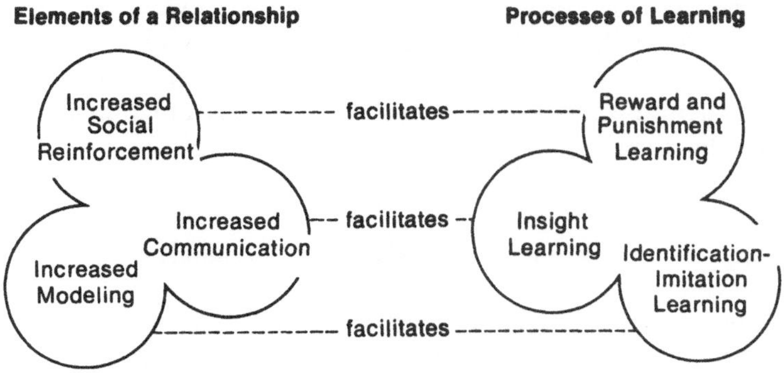

FIGURE 1: *How Relationship Facilitates Learning*

Figure 1 suggests how the existence of a "relationship" can strongly influence the child's learning, and thus his behavior. Each of the elements of a relationship facilitates modification of a child's behavior. The dotted lines indicate some of the more obvious ways that the relationship can be interrelated with learning. Thus, for example, if the child is responsive to the adult as a social reinforcer, then he is subject to influence by social approval and disapproval, and the adult is not restricted solely to using concrete rewards and punishments. If the child is receptive to communication with the adult, then he can be more easily influenced by the techniques of reasoning, explanation, suggestion or interpretation—techniques associated with insight learning. Finally, if the child chooses the adult as a model for his own behavior, then it is possible that the child will adopt a wide range of behaviors through identification with and imitation of the adult's behavior.

The foregoing sets the stage for our discussion of the practical considerations of relating therapeutically to disturbed and delinquent children. Whenever we speak of "establishing a relationship" we shall refer to (a) setting up communication with the child, (b) becoming significant enough to the child that the child will be responsive to adult approval or disapproval, and (c) providing an appropriate model for imitation. Our discussion will attempt to focus upon specific things the child-care worker can do—or avoid doing—to establish a "relationship beachhead." The invasion analogue of "beachheads" is not without relevance. It is perhaps most difficult to overcome the initial resistance of many of these children and to "get a hold" upon them; once we have "gotten through," we are then in a much better position to deploy our resources in the therapeutic service of the child.

Opening Communication Channels

Our previous discussion has suggested that an important aspect of developing relationships is in establishing and maintaining communication. Since communication is a two-way arrangement, we must be concerned with the content of two sets of "messages"—those we receive *from* the child and those we communicate *to* the child. These issues are discussed below under the headings "decoding the messages in behavior" and "communicating verbally and nonverbally."

Decoding the Messages in Behavior

It is important that the child-care worker develop some skill in understanding what children are saying, what they think, and how they feel. While this does not mean that he should become a "mind reader," it does suggest that he be sensitive to what the behavior of children can tell us about them. Perhaps this sensitivity is implicit in the personality of the worker and is not teachable. While a few individuals may never develop adequate sensitivity, it seems likely that most workers can become more perceptive of the messages conveyed by behavior.

The child-care worker is not a psychotherapist to the child, nor should he be. His main understanding of the child does not come from regular interviews as is the case in psychotherapy, but rather from the child's everyday behavior and natural conversation. Lest this sound like a skimpy basis for understanding the child, it should be remembered that most children tell us things about themselves in literally hundreds of ways every day. We learn about them in the way they greet us—the way they win, lose, succeed, fail, fight, withdraw, play, cry, eat, sleep, and so forth. It is unfortunate that those working directly with children often fail to decode the messages inherent in verbal and nonverbal behavior. The "on line" workers are usually so engrossed in problems of management that they fail to see what the behavior might mean.

Some might argue that the child-care worker is not capable of analyzing the child's behavior, since this requires considerable theoretical and clinical training. On the other hand, there is much that behavior can tell us, even if we do not resort to complicated theoretical schemes. We do not imply that it is desirable or even helpful for the worker to speculate about the distant roots of behavior; he should, however, realize that there is useful information communicated in the child's behavior, and to interact appropriately with the child we must first of all be able to "decode" the messages contained in his behavior.

The tricky part of this whole operation of "decoding" behavior is that these children often are experts in avoiding being "figured out." They have found it safest to conceal their real thoughts and feelings behind a diversionary front which serves to lead the observer off of the track. Thus, they may laugh when frightened or hurt, boast proudly when unsure, scowl angrily when pleased. If the worker is to communicate effectively with such children, he must develop an awareness of the sometimes subtle and partially hidden messages that are contained in the child's behavior.

It would be neither valuable nor possible to discuss all of the behavior that carries information about a child which might be useful to the child-care worker. It is possible, however, to consider two broad patterns of children's behavior which are very prevalent in residential treatment—patterns that often puzzle and confuse the worker. Perhaps if the worker better understands the meaning of such behavior, then he will be better able to react to the child in a manner that will foster the development of a positive relationship. The first of these behavior patterns we have called *orienting responses,* the reactions of the child to being placed in a new environment. The second pattern is referred to as interpersonal responses, that style of social behavior learned in the child's previous environment and now transferred to the new environment. Each of these will be discussed separately below.

Orienting Responses

Orienting responses are not unique to the new child entering a residential institution. Indeed, even adults engage in orienting behavior when they enter new and strange situations. The new situation is unpredictable: an individual does not know just how he should act, what the response of others will be, and what dangers might exist in this strange environment. In order to determine just what kind of place this is, the person engages in behavior aimed at orienting himself. By "orienting" we refer to (a) intense observing to gather clues about the unfamiliar situation, called *casing*, and (b) probing the environment to more fully examine uncertainties, called *limit testing*.

Casing. During the initial days or even weeks that the child is in residential treatment, he generally is involved in an information gathering operation which may be more picturesquely described as "casing the joint." He must become familiar with the physical facility, numerous peers, a large number of staff members—a considerable task to say the least. Redl and Wineman (1957) have described in detail how effective many of these youngsters are in determining the power structure of the group, assessing the delinquency proneness of peers, and determining the adult authority hierarchy. During this stage, many questions about rules, roles of different staff members, and who bosses them are apt to arise. Yet, since the adult is usually not trusted, the child will attach greater value to information he obtains from peers than that from adults. Child-care workers have sometimes found it useful to "arrange" the new child's initial peer contacts so that a more responsible youth is commissioned to "show him around." This makes it less likely that the newcomer will get negative information about the institution and the adults who work there.

Common sense and psychological research both attest to the

importance of "first impressions." While it may take months for people to learn what to expect from one another, much of this information is received in the initial encounter, and these impressions tend to color later judgments about the person. The significance of the initial encounter between worker and child should not be underestimated; children often remember vividly the first staff member they met upon arrival. The child is in a vulnerable position at this time; he has no real way of knowing what to expect, what you are like, what you might do to him, how he should deal with you. Since he may be entertaining negative expectations, a friendly encounter is indicated; however, this should have a businesslike air to it, since effusive warmth at this stage may only frighten him away or suggest to him that you are something of a mushy pushover. Our manner should communicate to the child that he is welcomed; that we look forward to working with him; that since he does not know us yet, we understand he is uncomfortable; and that he need not fear that we are going to harm him or push ourselves on him.

At the same time the child is casing our behavior, he is presenting a somewhat deceptive image of himself to others. Fearing that he will be set upon by others, he may begin by bragging about his prowess in this or that activity, be it slugging, sex, or swimming. The extent to which new children attempt to cover up their true self is seen in the following account of a new and frightened boy attempting to establish himself with those in his new environment:

> Randy was the loudest one before the swimming test. He bragged about how he had swum across a lake, could hold his breath three minutes under water, and had started to take lifesaving lessons. The other boys seemed impressed, and urged Randy to be the first boy to try the deep water test. Randy willingly complied, but it was a disaster. He dived [belly-flopped] into the water, came up choking. Even as he was being lifted from the water (rescued to be exact) he was still shouting, "The dock was slippery, let me try it again!" It was clear to both the campers and counselors that he couldn't swim a stroke.

During the initial days or weeks in residence, the child is apt to exhibit considerable restraint in his behavior. Not being sure what will happen to him, he manages to hold temporarily in check many of those behaviors that caused him to be sent into residential treatment. It is easy for the uninitiated adult to misconstrue an initially cooperative attitude as the beginning of a good relationship. In fact, this may often be only a "honeymoon" period that bears little resemblance to the more strained interactions that are to follow. For example, it is quite common for even extremely delinquent children to begin their interaction with the new adults in an overly polite "yes, sir—no, sir—whatever you say, sir" manner. The worker should not be fooled into concluding that this is the youngster's typical style of relationship, for the youth is apt to be fearful of the adult or may be attempting to deceive him. Unless the institution is one which demands that children always show "respect for elders," it is surprising how rapidly these "respectful" greeting styles disappear.

Limit testing. The child soon extends his orienting behavior beyond the casing stage: he begins to "test the limits." While he has learned a great deal by vicarious observation of peer behavior and adult response, he is usually compelled to engage in some personal limit testing himself. He seemingly must be certain what things he can get away with and what things bring some kind of reaction from the adult. Since several adults usually share in the task of managing him, he may "test out" each of them independently to determine who can control him and how they do it. At this point, the adult who was elated by the child's initial acquiescence may now feel that all has been lost. This is not so, but rather the child is only now beginning to act more "normally," and, in fact, this temporary behavior may be more extreme than his typical way of behaving.

The advent of testing behavior is particularly significant, since it signals that a real confrontation between the child and worker is imminent. Rather than flinch from this confrontation, the worker should look at this as an important opportunity to communicate to the child that he (the worker) is somehow different from many adults the child has previously encountered. Whether the adult handles this confrontation in a way that encourages further interaction or whether he alieniates the child remains to be seen.

Unlike his behavior of the first days of camp, Bob has been quite "testy" tonight. He intentionally tried to cause trouble after lights out by making anal noises. When we asked him to stop, he countered with, "What are you going to do if I don't?" We told him that he would have to leave the room if he couldn't keep still, and since he kept it up, we removed him (bodily). As he was struggling mildly, he suddenly grabbed my arm and asked, "Have you ever been bitten by a kid?" Somewhat startled, I tried to act calmly and answered, "Oh, a few times, I guess." He then asked what I would do if he bit me on the arm: "Would you belt me?" I told him that we don't hit kids here and don't expect that they will hurt grown-ups either. "But what *would* you do then, kick me out?" he continued. I told him that we didn't hurt kids and were not going to send him away, but that we "would think of something" if he acted like that. He was quiet for a couple of minutes, then said, "I am ready to go to sleep now." He sounded sincere, so I let him go back to the room and he caused no more problems.

The adult in the above situation apparently realized that the child was testing to determine what the limits for his behavior were—whether the adult could control him, and how the adult would exercise his control. It seems likely that this is part of the child's attempt to understand the conditions in his new environment. If such behavior can be handled in a straightforward, firm, but unexcited manner, the worker will not only weather this stage of the child's adjustment, but will achieve more status in the eyes of the child. If the worker becomes "rattled," unduly upset, or frightened by the negative behavior, the youngster will tend to devalue the competency of the adult and may even escalate his misbehavior until he can determine just where the limits are. If the adult overreacts with harsh punitive measures, this may have the detrimental side effect of lessening the tendency of the children to interact with the adult.

Particularly with the older youngster, the fact that the adult is able to "see through" and handle testing behavior can have a positive effect upon the development of a relationship, as suggested by the example below:

I went up to the cabin because the boys had been giving the

counselors a rough time and had balked at going to the afternoon activity. They were all lounging around on their beds. I had hardly started talking with them when Ray set me up by proclaiming, "We're all cutting out of here, going off grounds to get some weeds [cigarettes]." This was an announcement of two impending rule violations, and the boys waited intently to see how I would handle this. I shrugged my shoulders and said, "Well, the electric fence is turned off and the bloodhounds are on their day off; I guess today is as good a day as ever to get in trouble." The fellows all laughed, Ray smiled and said "You got cool man!" The tense atmosphere disappeared and our conversation turned to hot rods and the upcoming championship bout.

In the foregoing example, the worker sensed that his capacity to control the boys' prowess in a friendly and humorous manner had been tested. Had he been thrown off guard ("lost his cool" in the boys' vernacular), his status would have declined and the boys would perhaps have followed through on the threatened misbehavior. While a strong threat of reprimand might have deterred the announced incident (though it might have actually promoted it), it seems likely that this would have erected barriers between the boys and the worker.

How long do orienting responses, such as "limit testing," last? Usually after a few key confrontations such behavior diminishes, yet some children always seem to have a need to test the limits from time to time, no matter how long they have been in residential treatment. However, usually after the child has engaged in a period of testing behavior, he will settle into a pattern where he has everything pretty well figured out. He knows what to expect from the adults, and they know what to expect from him. When this orienting behavior diminishes, there is much less strain to interaction when it is prevalent, the adult must capitalize upon the confrontations, recognizing that he is laying the groundwork for what promises to be a more relaxed pattern of interaction between himself and the child.

We have discussed the child's reactions upon being placed in a new environment, referring to these behaviors as "orienting responses." We now shall consider the transfer of previously learned patterns of social behavior to the new environment.

We refer to these types of behavior as "interpersonal responses."

Interpersonal Responses [4]

There is a considerable body of evidence to suggest that the social behavior of an individual is characterized by consistent and stable tendencies to respond in particular ways to other persons.

This phenomenon has been referred to as a variety of terms (e.g., life style, life theme, interpersonal response traits), but the basic notion is actually relatively easy to understand:

> Each one of us . . . develops a distinctive set of enduring dispositions to respond to other people in characteristic ways. Thus one man will eye all of his neighbors as potential enemies and will be wary and suspicious in his dealings with them; another will see himself surrounded only by well-wishing friends and will be free and open in his social intercourse. These dispositions—here called *interpersonal response traits*— . . . help us to describe social man, to understand his behavior and to predict his actions (Krech, Crutchfield and Ballachey, 1962, p. 103).

While these interpersonal response "traits" or "styles" may result from constitutional as well as environmental factors, it appears that much of such behavior can be explained by a knowledge of how the individual perceives or interprets the social stimuli in his world. These perceptions have resulted from a lifetime of experience with many different people, the most significant of whom are usually the child's parents. Through all of his experience, the child has developed a set of expectations about people, and these expectations influence behavior. While there are numerous interpersonal response styles, we have selected out one as being particularly relevant to the child-care worker; this style is not descriptive of all children in residential treatment, but is extremely common

[4] Our discussion draws heavily on the concept of interpersonal response traits as discussed by Krech, Crutchfield, and Ballachey (1962) and upon the concept of life themes discussed by E. B. McNeil and R. L. Cutler (1966).

and presents sometimes baffling behavior to the worker. We have chosen to label this *the interpersonal response style of distrust.*

When the child leaves his former environment and is placed in a new situation, he brings along patterns of interpersonal response that appear to be inappropriate or maladaptive. One of the most common of such patterns of interpersonal behavior characteristic of children in residential treatment can be described in Erikson's (1963) terms of "basic mistrust." Unlike normal children, these children have not learned to associate adults with pleasant experiences; they have not found that adults meet their needs in predictable ways, nor can adults be counted on in time of trouble. More likely, they have learned that adults are connected with unpleasant circumstances, adults fail to provide what the child needs, and adults may even be dangerous to the child. The behavior of such children suggests that they view others with distrust, uncertainty, and suspicion.

When the child-care worker encounters such a child, the youngster does not suddenly discover that this adult is far different from other adults he has known. Rather, the child's interpersonal response style of distrust (learned over thousands of encounters with previous adults) stubbornly persists, even though (from the adults' viewpoint) it is no longer appropriate. Why does the child continue to misperceive the benign adult as if he were dangerous and not to be trusted? Since his perceptions are based on a lifetime of experience, he is unable to ignore suddenly all that he has previously learned just because the new adult acts somewhat differently from others he has known. This trait of distrust has served him well on numerous occasions when faced with a threatening or unpredictable adult; it is understandable why he will now tend to act toward the new adult in the same manner. From his point of view, it is likely that he is being deceived, and that beneath the friendly "front" of the adult is a person who, like others he has known, is not to be trusted. When the child-care worker tries to convince the child that he should trust the adult, the child is apt to become even more suspicious or frightened, and may develop strategies to "prove" that the adult cannot be trusted.

What are some of the strategies of behavior that are characteristic of *the interpersonal response style of distrust*? We discuss four categories of behavior below under the rubrics of "withdrawing," "disarming," "attacking," and "camouflaging."

Withdrawing. The simplest approach that the distrustful child might take is to avoid interaction with the adult. This is seen in his refusal to participate in activities with the adult, his avoidance of conversation, and in general by his total aloofness. To the child-care worker who is making conscientious attempts to draw the youngster into some kind of communication, such aloofness may be puzzling and discouraging. The new worker has not learned to have his attempts at reaching out to others meet with rebuff, and it is easy for him to respond to this frustration by abandoning efforts at communication with the child.

Ex. A. Whenever I would encounter Walter, I would greet him in a friendly manner. His response invariably was icy silence, coupled with turning his head away to avoid my glance. If I asked him anything, I was lucky to get even a grunt. This characterized our interaction for most of the winter, about three months.

Ex. B. Tony made it impossible to communicate with him, yet I felt that if I left him alone it would only reinforce his belief that we "didn't give a damn" about him. Finally we worked out a scheme where he was told, "We know you find it hard to say anything. However, since we like to talk with you, we will probably jabber a lot whenever we see you—you don't have to bother to answer us, though." Within a few days he became much more verbal.

Since withdrawal is a retreat from an undersirable situation, we must remember that we can make things worse by pursuing the child too closely. Very rarely is it indicated that we attack the child's withdrawal. Rather we would generally do better to approach him only cautiously, giving him time to become acquainted. We will consider this more fully later.

Disarming. Another way of handling someone that is a threat is to render the person harmless. In a sense, if the child "gets the upper hand," he need not fear the adult as strongly. These children develop an amazing repertoire of behaviors that serves to neutralize the effectiveness of the adult; this puts the adult on the defensive rather than the other way around. For example, the youngsters may claim that they "know something" about the worker and may even threaten to "tell the director all about it." At such a time, even the experienced worker finds himself thinking back to see what the kids might be referring to, if anything. The children are very sensitive to any behavior of the worker that could be held against him, and thus the worker will do well to quite rigorously observe high standards of language and conduct, lest the youngsters use the worker's behavior as a weapon against him. For example, one worker knew that several boys were smoking but yielded to their request that he not tell their therapists. Wanting to get on the good side of the boys, he agreed. Within a few days they were controlling him by threatening, "We'll tell the supervisor that you see guys smoking and don't do anything about it."

A similar defense against an adult is to strip him of his composure and competence, hoping that he will then retreat in fear. A good example of this is the behavior of two preadolescent boys toward a female worker, as described in the following manner:

> At dusk, Dale and Willy asked me if they could talk with me in "private like, outside on the steps." I was a little uncomfortable about this, but it looked like a good chance to communicate with them, so I agreed. They wanted to know what it was called when "a man does it to a lady to get babies," and I answered as frankly as I could. I soon discovered that I had walked into an ambush, since they were not interested in either information or technical terms, but were trying to get me to say the four-letter word which describes the process. When I wouldn't say it, they shifted to accusing me of having had intercourse with Walter [another counselor] and said that someone had reported seeing us "in the bushes" the

night before. I was so rattled that I said, "Well, it must have been someone else because it wasn't Walter and me," which was certainly not the right thing to say. I cut off the discussion, but every time they would see me they would call me a "whore"; I finally had to get the supervisor to talk to them about this name calling. It stopped but they then shifted to making sly references about the supervisor and me.

Another common way that distrustful children employ to neutralize the efforts of the child-care worker is to view him as having other motives instead of his supposedly therapeutic interest in the children. Thus, the worker is accused of "only doing this because of the money" or of "doing this because he couldn't get any other job" or "he would beat us except he is afraid he'll get fired." This gives the child a way of holding to his life style of distrust of adults, even though the worker may not act the same way other adults have acted.

Attacking. If the child's experiences have taught him that adults are dangerous and should not be trusted, then he is apt to be somewhat confused when his experiences with the child-care worker do not bear this out. He may try to prove that the adult is untrustworthy in a number of ways. One of the most common is to "catch" the adult in a lie: it is not unusual for the worker, even though he strictly observes the principle of never lying to the child, to find that the children will search for picayunish flaws in his statements, which then "prove" the adult's unreliability. Yet, if the worker has handled these situations sensibly, the child may have to resort to cruder methods of establishing the adult's untrustworthiness. The most extreme method is to provoke a fight with an adult.

Gary was upset with the way his counselor, Hal, had called one of the plays in the baseball game. When they went back up to the cottage, he persisted in a stream of profanity directed at Hal. When this did not evoke any equivalent response from Hal, Gary walked up to Hal, and in a nonimpulsive, calculated manner began to kick Hal in the shins. Hal tried to joke with him to get him to stop, but Gary persisted. Whereupon Hal (finally becoming angry at this assault) gave Gary a push to get him away from him. Though he obviously hadn't been hurt, Gary began to scream almost hysterically at Hal, then ran from the cottage, sobbing that he would never come back. Another worker had to retrieve Gary since he actually was running away. When he was brought back by the second counselor he persisted in the theme that Hal tried to beat him up.

The foregoing is an extreme example, but it does suggest that a child may arrange it so that the adult's response reinforces his distorted perception of adults. Generally the child will not provoke an attack on himself in such a straightforward way. It is very common, however, for children to threaten verbally or insult an adult; if the adult responds to this as a challenge to battle, he will only reinforce the child's life theme of distrust. On the other hand, one must do something, and it is not necessarily the best thing to always ignore the provocation, as the following child-care worker mistakenly believed:

> When I told Rodney that he had to go to bed, he refused. I insisted, and to my surprise, he slapped me on the face. I told him he couldn't make me angry, so I turned my cheek, whereupon he slapped me on the other side of my face. I then calmly walked away.

It is not necessary that we communicate that we can never be angered or provoked, for with most of us such passivity under attack is almost impossible. Yet, in the way that we respond to the child, we must avoid giving him fuel for his notion that we are like the other dangerous or distrustful adults he has encountered. This topic will be considered again when we discuss management of the upset child (Chapter VII).

Camouflaging. We have seen how distrustful children cope with adults by utilizing strategies of withdrawing, disarming, or attacking. These strategies usually prevent the development of a positive relationship, since the natural reactions of the adult tend to reinforce the child's distrust. But, even if the adult is able to cope effectively with the child's defensive strategies, the child is rarely able to abandon suddenly his established response style of distrust. As the child begins to engage cautiously in more trustful interactions, he often disguises his emerging interest in the adult under the cloak of his old style of behavior. The following example illustrates this; the worker fortunately was able to detect the beginnings of a positive relationship even though the child's interest in the worker was camouflaged by hostile behavior.

> Every day when I would come on duty at 3:30, Jim would just "happen" to be waiting around. He would always greet me with a comment like, "Oh, hell! Look who we have to put up with tonight." Or "Here comes the worst counselor we have!" Or he would groan and tell me how much he hated me. I always countered with a friendly greeting, having the feeling that he really didn't mind me that much, although he never greeted the other counselors the same insulting way. Then one day he gave himself away: "I can hardly wait until December, fourth, fifth, eighth, and eleventh when you will have your days off." Since the work schedule constantly changes (and I have enough trouble myself remembering my days off), it became clear that he had made a special effort to know when I wouldn't be at work. "I guess I'll miss you, too, on my days off," I replied. He smiled sheepishly, but from that day his greetings gradually started getting friendlier; he would still insult me, but would punctuate it with a friendly smile.

Another variation of camouflaged behavior is that of children who use rough physical means of communication with the adult. They may jump aggressively on his back, punch him on the arm, take something of his and run, etc. Such behavior is generally the child's way of initiating interaction, and the adult who deals harshly with this is actually punishing social interaction as much as the specific objectionable behavior. The best response will be one that communicates to the child that the adult likes to have fun with him, but that there are better ways of having fun than that which he has chosen.

It would be too much of a radical change from his interpersonal style if all of a sudden the distrustful child treated adults in a trusting manner. By camouflaging his interest in the adult under seemingly hostile or frivolous behavior he can both maintain some communication and further test out the safety of the adult. If the adult misinterprets the child's behavior he may cause the child to abandon further communication. The situation is not unlike that of the early adolescent boy who, not having learned to be comfortable with girls, expresses his interest in them by teasing them. The smart little girls learn to play along with the teasing so that the interaction keeps going. Other girls tell the teacher, frighten the boy away, and grow up without boyfriends.

Communicating Verbally and Nonverbally

Communicating Verbally

Each day the child-care worker has hundreds of opportunities to communicate verbally with his charges, even though the topics of conversation are at times unexciting and the presence of the group precludes a great deal of individual conversation. Among different workers, there is a wide range in the ability to communicate with disturbed children. While certain workers seem always to have a group of children gathered about them involved in some discussion, other workers are clearly uncomfortable whenever they are talking to or listening to a child. This tension is most noticeable with new workers who often express their concern by questions such as "How do you involve them in a conversation?" or "What do you talk about with them?" In this section we shall attempt to point out some guidelines and pitfalls of talking with disturbed children.

Verbal communication is much easier in some situations than in others. For example, certain table games are almost always accompanied with conversation that may or may not be related to the activity itself. The activity provides the structure for communication that would otherwise be difficult or impossible. Even as adults, we find it difficult to engage in conversation without the benefit of "props," unless we know the other person quite well. Thus, we have bridge clubs, poker parties, golf games, and sewing bees, all of which facilitate communication between the participants. This is an important principle for the child-care worker to remember, since much of his initial communication with the children can be structured by the activities and routines of cottage life.

But if communication never went beyond the "bridge conversation" stage, it is unlikely that the worker will find the children eager to talk with him. While just being a "good listener" will draw certain children to him, with most youngsters he will have to take a considerably more active role. In the initial stages of a relationship, the worker who can engage freely in "small talk" or light humor will be at a decided advantage. Much of the social interaction that exists in adult society is of this caliber. Lest the reader becomes indignant at our prescription of "small talk," we hasten to emphasize that this is the means to an end, not an end itself. Unfortunately, some adults and children are never able to get beyond this stage in their communication.

The topic of conversation is a crucial variable in the establishment and maintenance of communication. What does one talk about with disturbed and delinquent children? This is a very puzzling question to many adults who can think of nothing to ask a child beyond his name and age. The answer depends upon the age, sex, and background of the child, and it is hard to prescribe specific topics. Effective workers take their cues from what the children talk about on their own and what the child seems to be interested in. Thus, even as we help a new child move into a cottage, we can get cues by noting what he brings with him: unfortunately it sometimes happens that a worker will unpack a child's swimming suit, snorkel, skin-diving magazines, and deep sea adventure comics without knowing what to talk about with him.

Certain topics have higher probabilities of being interesting to the child. For example, football, boxing, drag racing, hot rods, guns, the latest musical groups—these are likely to interest most boys. The worker should expect that he may be encountering an expert on one of these topics, and if the worker tries to sound "in" by endorsing the "Four Seasons," he may find that what he thought was the latest musical group is now "out of season." Some workers have found it is helpful to try to keep abreast of the developments in some of these fields (even when they are not personally interested in the subject) to avoid becoming a "conversational dropout."

For some reason, many workers feel that their interaction with disturbed children is not really "therapeutic" unless they are talking about the child's "conflicts" or problems. It should be emphatically stated that many of the workers who have the most positive effect upon the children they handle do so without ever opening up issues of a "psychological" nature. In fact, it is often contraindicated for workers to engage in this sort of amateur psychotherapy role. The following examples should illustrate some of these problems.

We were warned by the state hospital that the first thing Jim would try to do is to "get an audience" for his tales of woe. This was particularly dangerous, since he had a habit of talking himself into a very depressed state and had actually attempted suicide in such a situation. We thought we had warned everybody to change the topic if he started out on his problems, but nobody remembered to tell the social group work student. Sure enough, first thing we knew he was up in a tree, threatening to jump, with the student trying to talk him down. He had started talking to her about how his parents hated him. She thought she was getting some important information and led him on, and got over her head. We had her leave, and in a couple of minutes the supervisor was able to "talk him down."

Tony had been talking with Fred (counselor) about home trouble with his parents, etc., most every night before bedtime. When the midnight staff would come on duty, Tony would still be restless, complaining that he didn't feel good and couldn't get to sleep.

Bill developed a good relationship with his child-care counselor, Ed, and started to tell Ed all of the things that he told his doctor in the therapy session. As Ed encouraged this, Bill brought up more and more hithertofore unknown things about his previous background. But, simultaneously as he began to communicate about all of this highly personal data with Ed, he quit talking in his psychotherapy sessions. It got so that the only way the therapist could find out anything about Bill was to ask the counselor, and finally the counselor had to be told to discontinue his discussions; Bill began to "produce" in therapy again.

These examples illustrate how the child-care worker who sees his role as that of psychotherapist can quickly find himself in a situation he is unable to handle. This does not mean that the worker must *never* talk with the youngster about problems, only that he should be careful what sort of problems he discusses. A good rule of thumb is to keep things geared to the present situation, i.e., the difficulties encountered in the living situation and in peer interaction, but to avoid discussion of the child's background or family situation. Rather than being hamstrung, the worker will find that there are more than enough immediate, everyday problems which need attention without digging back into the child's case history. If the child persists in initiating discussions the worker does not feel capable of handling, a tactful referral is indicated.

If the child thinks that the worker is "zeroing in" on his personal problems, it is not unusual for him to become frightened. Some youngsters suspect that everybody in the place is something of a "head shrinker" in disguise, and the worker who places himself in this role will only drive these suspicious children from him. The extreme sensitivity of the sophisticated delinquent to this issue is illustrated in the following description of a counselor's conversation with an 11-year-old youngster:

> I was standing by the waterfront, visiting with Mac about canoeing, fishing, and things in general. As Mac seemed very open and communicative, I suggested that instead of standing we "go sit down on that log over there." He gave me a funny look and said, "Oh, no you don't! You can't pull any of that psychology stuff on me!" He turned and walked away, avoiding me the rest of the day.

Everybody uses some amount of "small talk" and standard greetings to lessen the anxiety in brief encounters with others. Since many of these children are unusually uncomfortable in any conversation with adults, it is sometimes helpful if the adult limits his early interactions to short and brief exchanges. Normal cottage life gives the child-care worker numerous chances to "happen by" in the course of a given day, and it may be to the worker's advantage if he can "program" small doses of interaction, perhaps of only a few seconds duration; these seem not to be anxiety producing and thus, do not produce withdrawal behavior. For example, a worker who is slowly developing communication with a particular youth meets him on the sidewalk; deciding it would be too threatening to the boy to "stop and talk," but wishing to communicate beyond a simple greeting, he may say, "Here comes that fellow who beat me in basketball yesterday." The boy says nothing, but smiles as he recalls having beat the counselor 20 to 18 in a game the day before. It is likely that communication will be a bit less inhibited the next time they meet.

Just because a child is interested in a particular topic of conversation does not mean that that will be a good thing to talk about. Experienced workers with disturbed children have learned that there are certain recurring topics of discussion that need to be labelled as "handle with care." Thus the worker should sense when he is being set up as the straight man for an off-color joke: If he is asked if he knows what the farmer said to the traveling salesman when such and such happened, it might be wise for the worker to smoothly disengage himself from the conversation, perhaps with a comment like, "You guys are just being silly." Likewise, the worker becomes cautious when the youngsters ask certain questions about his personal life. While this may be only a legitimate interest in the adult, it is often something of a "trap." It is unwise to discuss early delinquencies of the worker, though the children may ask if he ever got kicked out of school, or was arrested, or stole something. The children are certain to ask if the worker is married, which merits a truthful response; however, this is often the lead-in to more probing questions (e.g., "Then, do you have a steady girl friend?"), and the worker must be prepared to disentangle himself from the discussion before he is asked something too personal. The worker should not feel obligated to bring his personal life out for the children to examine, but rather to be free to change the topic or parry the question in the smoothest way possible. The alternative is to risk being dragged in deeper than one should go.

Talking is not always a pleasant thing. The worker will engage in considerable communication at times when the child is in open defiance, and some very barbed comments are sometimes directed at the worker. All workers are pushed near their explosion point at times, and it takes considerable self-control, experience, and perhaps humor before the worker learns how to respond at these times. Sometimes the worker will find that he is so angry that he is unsure of what he might say or how his voice will sound if he opens his mouth; he might do better to maintain silence for a little while, remembering that one can always say something later but it is not possible to retrieve the spoken word once said. If he can refrain from saying something, he has a chance to recollect his thoughts and may even think of something sensible to say or do. Likewise, if the child is extremely angry, it is sometimes better if the worker waits a bit before attempting to communicate with the child. There are ways, however, of neutralizing the child's anger, and we will consider these more fully in Chapter VII.

We have stressed that the worker should take cues for conversation from the interests of the child. It is likewise possible for the worker to bring his own hobbies, interests, or ideas into the conversation, and some children might be quite interested in these. There is a caution in this, however. Workers sometimes bring up topics that are not appropriate for consumption by the children. Many child-care workers are associated with college student populations in which there are strong feelings about free speech and broad tolerance for deviant ideas. It is necessary that the worker adequately separate his personal philosophy of life from his work with children, particularly if his ideas are controversial. Disturbed children have enough to worry about without wrestling with the same conflicts facing the worker. We refer specifically to such issues as religion, politics, sexual morality, civil rights, etc. While the worker may have very strong feelings on some of these issues, he must exercise considerable discretion; he is working with children rather than adults and somebody else's children at that.

Communicating Nonverbally

Behavioral scientists have been studying nonverbal communication for nearly four decades, but as of yet our knowledge is only very fragmentary. Even a tiny child can decode the messages in the expressive behavior or "body language" of his parents (Sullivan, 1953), yet research has only begun to speculate about what is actually going on, e.g., what cues the child is using. Although there is as yet little scientific basis to our discussion of this topic, we still feel compelled to point out some of the hunches we have about the role of nonverbal behavior in communication with disturbed children.

Our discussion assumes that (a) children attach meaning to much of our nonverbal behavior, (b) that certain behaviors tend to be perceived in more or less standard ways, and (c) that the child-care worker is capable of controlling or modifying some of his nonverbal behavior in order to communicate appropriate messages to the child. The following two hypothetical examples will illustrate what we mean:

A youth openly defies his worker's demand that he go to his room. The worker, sensing the impending confrontation approaches the youngster with "hands ready" in a manner like that sketched here; the child lunges at the worker.

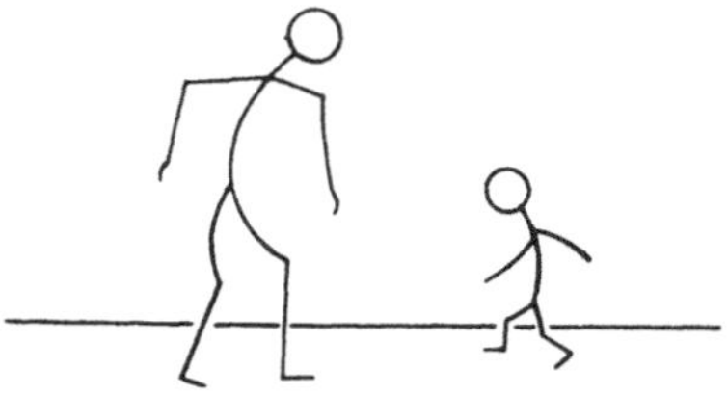

The same youth openly defies his worker's demand that he go to his room. The worker, although sensing an impending confrontation, approaches the youngster in a relaxed manner as sketched here; the child grumbles but complies.

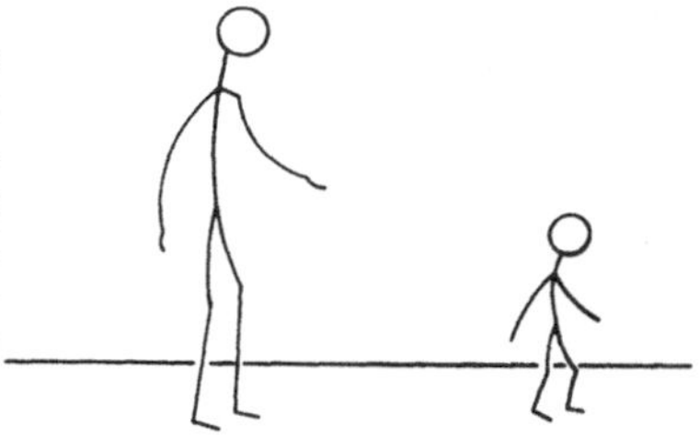

In the first example, the worker communicated by his stance that he expected trouble and was prepared to use force. In the second example, the worker communicated through his relaxed stance that he did not expect any trouble, but assumed that the child would comply. We suggest that the youngster might respond in different ways, depending upon the nonverbal message he receives.

We may be surprised to discover that there is a great deal of nonverbal communication among humans, since our verbal proficiency sometimes causes us to overlook the importance of nonverbal channels. Even animals respond differently to one another on the basis of the posture one animal takes when encountering another animal; there are certain threatening postures (e.g., the cat with arched back), as well as nonthreatening postures (e.g., in many species the animal rolls over on his back, exposing his vital parts to the other and assuming a vulnerable position). What are some examples of nonverbal communication that are important to the child-care worker?

We have suggested that certain postures signal when trouble is imminent. Many child-care workers have the habit of communicating "imminent attack" to children by their stance, their tone of voice, or other cues; such workers usually do not have the slightest idea what it is about them that causes their almost constant conflict with aggressive children. In contrast, other workers do not assume such threatening stances, but are more likely to employ nonverbal communication in a number of positive ways. They may use eye contact, nods of the head, gestures, physical proximity to communicate to the child (without words) that he is understood, or that he has just done something well, or that we will help him control himself or protect him, and so forth. Such is the case in the following account by a child-care worker:

> Rodney had been discharged from the training school, but after only four days at home he was apprehended by the police for molesting a young girl. He was returned to the school and brought to the cottage where I was on duty. I could tell that he wondered if I "knew" and if I still liked him, as he stayed aloof in the corner of the room and appeared to be crying. I couldn't think of anything to say, so I just ambled over to him and very lightly "punched" him on the arm. He looked up through his tears and said, "Thanks. I wish my old man understood like you."

Children are very attuned to nonverbal cues; the worker will discover that the youngsters detect feelings he is not even aware of himself. One of the authors recalls a situation some years ago when the group was challenging his authority; at the point when the author's patience was almost exhausted, one of the youngsters suddenly exclaimed, "Oh, oh! Better watch out, he's whistling again, he must be getting mad!" Sure enough, although not aware of it, he later noted that whenever he was reaching his "breaking point" he started whistling.

Children are also very perceptive of the nonverbal "asides" which workers give one another as they share the task of dealing with difficult clients; if two workers exchange nervous smiles when a child does something devious, they should expect that the youngster will also note this behavior.

It is not possible to go into all of the nuances of nonverbal communication; nonverbal communication is not a few isolated techniques, it is an entire language, and a language for which no dictionaries have yet been compiled. But we do suggest that the worker become aware of the importance of the nonverbal communication that develops between himself and the children. In the following discussion we shall consider certain common cautions the child-care worker should display with respect to one variety of nonverbal communication: physical contact.

Physical Contact. Few issues are the source of so much concern and yet receive so little discussion as does physical contact between worker and child. The child-care worker is variously advised (a) that physical contact is his most important means of communication with many children, (b) that physical contact should be used only sparingly and discretely, or (c) that physical contact should be avoided if at all possible. The worker is warned about being "seductive," yet he finds it difficult and unnatural to live in close proximity with the children and still keep them "at arm's length." Many highly effective workers feel that the physical gestures they utilize in their work with disturbed children are indispensable in establishing relationships.

While it may seem that physical contact would create problems only when male workers interact with girls or female workers with boys, this is not the case. Neither is the confusion about the role of physical contact exclusive to the new and inexperienced worker. While the issue of physical contact may be of particular relevance in work with adolescents, the problem is not restricted to interactions with older children. Lurking unspoken beneath these concerns is the possibility that some workers may be seeking their own personal gratification through excessive use of physical contact. This need not imply anything so drastic as "illicit" physical contact, but pertains to the more common situation where the worker constantly "hovers" over certain children, finds almost any pretext for putting his or her arm around the child, or engages in much physical horseplay such as tickling or wrestling. The main thing that can be wrong with such contact is that it appears to be motivated primarily out of the worker's own needs, rather than what is appropriate to the particular child at a given time.

Yet there are several reasons why physical contact may be effective in establishing relationships with certain children. Since many maladjusted youngsters respond only minimally to verbal means of communication, physical contact provides a ready nonverbal channel. There is some evidence that children from lower class backgrounds tend to be more physically expressive than verbally expressive (McNeil, 1960), and to be more attuned to nonverbal cues than verbal cues (Manuchin, 1966). Research with animals suggests that physical contact is the primary factor in the formation of attachments between individuals (Harlow, 1960). Indeed, physical contact is invariably present in the most intimate of human relationships (mother-child, husband-wife). It is not unrealistic, then, to expect that some physical contact would be a natural element in relationship formation, particularly with younger children.

Physical contact can be employed to convey to a child feelings that cannot be easily put into words or that would sound inappropriate if verbalized. For example, the child-care worker who responds to a child's friendly greeting by tussling the youngster's hair might have difficulty if he employed an equivalent verbalization, such as "I'm glad to see you and I like you!" But, using physical contact as a technique in building relationships with disturbed children is tricky business, as the new worker soon discovers. There are definite situations in which any type of physical contact would be contraindicated, and there are many different types of physical contact. Therefore, the child-care worker should be aware of the following cautions, presented not as arguments against physical contact *per se*, but as factors which must be considered if the worker is to utilize physical contact appropriately.

Physical Contact and Peer Rivalry. Physical contact sometimes backfires if it occurs in a visible situation where it can be noted by other children. Many disturbed children have very little ability to share an adult with others, and the mere sight of the worker giving physical contact to one child often evokes strong feelings of jealousy and competition in other children. This is particularly true if the worker is generally well liked by the children. Since the worker is simultaneously concerned with developing or maintaining relationships with several different children, he must avoid upsetting or even alienating one child by the attention he gives another. Such a problem is exemplified in the following report by a child-care worker:

> As the group was walking from the ball field, Terry jumped up on my back and asked for a "piggy-back ride." My usual response in such a situation is to ease the kid off my back, jokingly groaning that he is too big and heavy and so should walk beside me. Since this was the first time Terry had shown any sign of acting in a friendly way toward me, I decided to give him a ride. When we got up to the cottage, the others all demanded rides too, particularly Alvin who was almost crying as he exclaimed, "You never give me a ride. . . . you like Terry better than me!"

In such a situation as described above, the child-care worker must be able to say no to the child who is seeking excessive physical contact, and yet avoid the possibility that the child would interpret this as rejection.

Physical Contact and Sexual Stimulation. Physical contact which seems very innocent may become highly stimulating to some disturbed children. This is a potential problem regardless of the sex and age of the child or of the worker. These children are frequently unable to deal with their aroused emotions in an appropriate manner, and may respond with anxiety or guilt, with aggression, or with other undesirable behavior. The following examples illustrate this:

Ex. A: Tyrone (age 11) approached the supervisor and said that he had a problem. Could the supervisor tell Mary (his counselor) to stay away from his bed after he gets in his pajamas?

"She gets me all turned on when she stoops over like that and tucks me in, and I can't get to sleep thinking about her."

Ex. B: Barbara (counselor) asked that I talk with Robert (age 12) about keeping his hands off her. She reported that he would start by holding her hand or putting his hand on her shoulder, and then his hands would start to stray. If she tried to stop him, he would become angry and slap at her. When Robert was confronted with this behavior, he became quite angry and claimed, "She puts her hands on me, so why can't I put mine on her too." We worked out an agreement where nobody would put their hands on anybody else.

A few disturbed children are so readily stimulated that it is necessary to maintain a total "hands off" policy. For example, in one situation an adolescent with a history of homosexual encounters with older men seemed to welcome physical gestures. It was decided that the male workers should avoid any physical contact in their interactions with him. Such an arrangement can prove difficult if the child persists in forcing physical contact. This is perhaps best exemplified in the case reported by McDermott, Fraiberg, and Harrison (1966) in which an adolescent boy derived sexual satisfaction from being physically restrained during periods of uncontrolled behavior.[5]

Physical Contact as an Anxiety Producing Stimulus. A further caution concerning the use of physical contact is that certain youngsters, because of their past experiences, have learned that physical contact may signal some kind of threat to them. The child who is fearful of developing relationships with others because of past rejection may be frightened by the intimacy of physical contact. Sometimes a child who has been subjected to extreme brutality may "cringe" or "tense up" when an adult touches him, seemingly expecting attack even in the gesture of a friendly hand on his shoulder. Other disturbed children with unusual sexual histories may misinterpret even the most innocuous physical contact as a sexual advance; they may project their own problem on the worker, accusing him or her

[5] The issue of physical contact during periods of physical restraint will be considered further in Chapter VII.

of being "queer" or of being "a whore." Finally, there are certain children who have obsessive fantasies about what might happen to them if others touch them; such a case was reported by Rubin (1961) in *Lisa and David.* Fortunately this latter disorder is very rare.

Physical Contact and Aggression. It is quite common for male child-care workers to employ "rough and tumble" procedures in their relationships with boys. They may engage in physical horseplay, participate in contact sports like football or wrestling, or otherwise engage the youngsters in a physical manner. Some workers feel that it is essential that they establish their physical superiority over the child if they are to control and relate positively to him. Yet, while some degree of physical testing of the worker is sometimes necessary, there is a real danger that the adult will slip into an aggressive role not unlike that occupied by former, sometimes brutal adults that the children have known. While it may initially seem that the only thing the boys will respect is physical force, yet if physical force is employed in even a slightly hostile manner, the child may over-react in a negative manner. Even "good rough fun" may produce this effect as illustrated by the following:

> Essex refused to go into the cottage after the evening swim. When pressure was applied, he became tearful, saying "I won't go in the same room with Ralph [counselor]as long as I live! He tried to kill me under the water." We called Ralph over to discuss the incident. It seemed that all that happened was that Ralph was a little overly eager in horseplay with the boys in the water. Essex apparently choked on some water, and assumed Ralph was trying to drown him. Ralph apologized to Essex, assuring him that he hadn't meant to hurt him, and Essex finally went into the cottage.

As a general rule of thumb, it is probably best to avoid activity where it is easy for the worker to hurt a youngster. What seems to be innocent fun to the worker can readily become a physical attack when viewed from the perspective of the child who distrusts adults.

With all of the problems that can result, might it not be best to eliminate any type of physical contact? Perhaps this *is* the best approach in some situations, as in work with adolescents, particularly when female workers deal with boys or male workers with girls. Yet, in many situations the worker would be unwise to abandon the careful use of physical contact as an important instrument in establishing relationships with disturbed or delinquent children.

Increasing Interpersonal Attraction

Our previous discussion focused on the communication between worker and child. In this section of the chapter, we shift our discussion to issues of particular relevance to becoming a positive social reinforcer and an appropriate behavioral model for the child. But, we must preface our remarks with a caution. We really do not understand all of the reasons why a child strives to obtain the approval of particular adults, nor why he elects to model the behavior of some adults and not of others. We would expect that a child would be highly motivated to obtain the approval of a benign parent, yet a child may strive equally as hard to obtain the approval of a rejecting parent. Likewise, a child may not only model his parents' behavior, but also that of perfect strangers. Until further research clarifies these issues, no single explanation seems adequate.

Though our understanding of these issues is inadequate, the child-care worker is still faced with the problem of trying to establish his value to the child as a social reinforcer and a behavior model. There is some research that suggests that the more favorably the child regards the adult, the more receptive he will be to the adult's influence (Goldstein, Heller and Sechrest, 1966). It might be expected that such influence might occur through the processes of reward-punishment learning (i.e., social reinforcement) and identification-imitation learning, as well as through insight learning.

Our discussion is organized around the topic of "increasing interpersonal attraction." If a child is not attracted to an adult (does not view the adult favorably), he is less responsive to the adult's influence attempts; such is the case with many disturbed and delinquent children. It seems possible to attempt to alter the situation in three ways. First, the positive attributes of the adult may be emphasized or increased. Second, the negative attributes may be minimized or eliminated. Third, since the child is more attracted to (or less repelled by) the adult at certain times (such as time of crisis), the adult can capitalize on these periods when the child is most tractable. Each of these three approaches is discussed below.

Maximizing Adult Attractiveness

How does the child-care worker increase his attractiveness to the disinterested child? First, the fact that the worker is involved in dispensing a certain amount of concrete gratifications to the child tends to increase his importance to the child. Some theories of residential treatment place a great deal of emphasis upon the importance of gratifying the needs of the child. While total gratification is neither practical nor theoretically sound, the fact remains that if the adult is associated with positive situations (need satisfaction), then he will tend to acquire positive characteristics to the child. In many institutions the adults are rarely associated with positive situations (at least in comparison to the frequency with which they are associated with negative situations), and it is easy to understand why the children do not find the adults to be very attractive.

However, the worker will usually have to provide considerably more than satisfaction of basic needs if he is to become attractive to the child. One way he can do this is through activities. The worker must ask two questions: first, what is already important to the child, attracts him, or is desired by him? Second, what special skills, talents, or ideas do I have that might be of interest to the child? Since children and child-care workers are both very diverse groups of individuals, a wide variety of activities may suggest themselves.

It is surprising how certain activities will capture the interest of one youngster, and yet be ignored or despised by others. While a worker might find that his swimming skill provides the basis for his attractiveness to one youngster, it will be his guitar playing that draws another child's interest. Our observations indicate that the attraction of children to different workers has been based on such diverse worker skills as campcraft, auto mechanics, gardening, sewing, art, music, foreign languages, model airplanes, stamp collecting, fishing, and even bee-keeping. In each case, the worker shared an interest with the child, or possessed a skill the child wished to obtain. In general, the more skills available to the worker, the greater probability that he will be attractive to a particular child. Just what skill may not be so important, as long as there is *some* answer to the implicit question of the youngsters, "so, what's so good about him!" The importance should not be underestimated, and Chapter III is devoted to a consideration of how to program activities for individuals and groups.

Other things besides activities are important to children. For example, Kvaraceus and Miller (1959) talk of several focal concerns common in the lower class subculture including such things as toughness, excitement, and smartness. It seems likely that the adult who is seen to possess these attributes might be viewed more favorably by some youth than the adult who was viewed as weak, colorless, and gullible. In the eyes of many delinquents, smartness is not measured in academic degrees. Rather, it refers to a person's ability to handle people and situations and to avoid being "conned" by others. Likewise, many delinquent children seem to be attracted to novel, unexpected, and exciting stimuli; the adult who interacts in novel, sometimes unpredictable ways may be more attractive to such a youngster.

With some children, it is necessary that the worker establish that no matter what the child might do, in the long run the adult has the upper hand and cannot be manipulated or deceived. With these highly controlling and manipulative children, the only way the adult may be able to establish his value for the child is to surpass him at his own game. Clinical experience indicates that these children typically evoke one of two types of response from the adult. Either the adult allows himself to be overpowered by the child, or the adult employs severe sanctions on the child. In both cases, the attractiveness of the adult diminishes since the child perceives him as weak and ineffective, or as hostile and unfair. A third alternative is available to the adult, and has the advantage that the adult neither capitulates nor utilizes excessively aversive control techniques; he merely outmaneuvers the child. Two examples of such situations are given below; both occurred with the same worker and child.

Rod (age 12) was angry when the counselor insisted that he had to take his shower like the other boys before he could join in the evening snack. "If I can't have my Kool-Aid right now, nobody else will either!" he exclaimed. He calmly walked to the dining room table, spit in the pitcher of beverage, and strode from the room with the satisfaction that he had shown the worker who was boss. Before the other boys had time to react, the worker announced (loudly enough so Rod could hear), "Dump out the Kool-Aid, boys; tonight we'll get ice cream." Rodney began cursing, ran down to his room, and cried for a while, then took his shower and caused no further problems that evening.

Rod knew he was in trouble for fighting with Tony. When the counselor sought him out, he was perched atop the cottage roof, declaring that if anyone wanted to talk with him, they would have to come up and get him off the roof. The counselor, apparently not relishing the notion of a wrestling match on the roof-top, told him that no matter how long he stayed up there, he will still have to settle the fight problem when he came down. "Well, we'll just see who can wait the longest!" Rod exclaimed. "You can wait, but I have work to do," said the worker, and he started to walk away. Rod then began hollering to the others to join him on the roof. The counselor countered by telling the other members of the group, "Last one to the gym is *it* for dodge ball!" Everyone left the scene following the counselor; in about a half hour Rod came to the gym and told the counselor he was "ready to talk."

Contrary to expectations, being able to control a manipulative child does not alienate him, if the control is exercised in a basically nonpunitive manner. Hoffer (1949) and Aichhorn (1935) have both written of the utility of being able to outsmart the child who feels he can manipulate or deceive most adults. In a sense, the worker beats the child at his own game. Since what is important to the youth is the ability to manipulate others, the adult with sufficient prowess who avoids being manipulated is in possession of an attribute which the youth desires. We both caution the worker who is employing techniques to outmanipulate the child that the adult manipulation must occur within the framework of socially acceptable behavior; this rules out such adult techniques as deliberately lying to a youngster. Furthermore, it should be clear that the relationship must proceed beyond the initial stage of a young con artist admiring an older, more experienced one.

Approaches to Avoid. In the effort to increase their attractiveness to the child, workers sometimes employ approaches which backfire in one way or the other. Four such errant approaches are commonly observed. The first of these is the erroneous assumption of the worker that if he will "be easy on the kids," they will like him more. The youngsters themselves sometimes supply fuel to this assumption by their threat that they won't ever talk to the adult again if he doesn't do such and so. The worker, aware that many of the youngsters have known inconsistent and brutal administration of adult controls, may assume that a permissive and totally accepting attitude will be the best approach. While this may be all right in individual psychotherapy it can only lead to trouble in the group living situation. Most of the children need external controls, may even ask for them, and will view the worker who never interferes as being frightened and inadequate.

Another error made by new workers is to attempt to "become one of the boys." This is common among younger workers (e.g., college students) who have not yet fully adopted the adult role themselves, and who may find it more natural to act as a member of the youngster's peer group. While younger workers can be particularly effective with many children since they do not engender the distrust that is harbored toward adults, it is essential that the worker carve out some sort of adult role. Sooner or later he will be forced into precarious control situations that will make him wish he had a different role with the group. Furthermore, the biggest lesson that many of these children need to learn is how to relate to adult authority figures: the worker who disavows this role removes the possibility that the child will learn this from him.

A third error made by workers is to build up his attractiveness by criticizing other adults the child knows. The worker may disalign himself with the administrative or supervisory staff or with other workers by telling the child, "I am different from them." He may even attempt to contrast himself with the child's own parents, perhaps the most serious error he can make. Children who were unable to function in foster homes often report that the foster parent kept reminding them about "how much better treatment we are giving you than your parents provided." Tearing down others on the staff disrupts the functioning of the program; tearing down a child's parents (even if he himself says negative things about them) is the supreme insult, no matter how subtly it is done.

The fourth error sometimes made by the child-care worker is to "become the child's new parent." This is also labeled overinvolvement, and it refers to the very real problem that some workers overdo their efforts to become attractive to the child. We cannot promise to be all things to a child unless that child is our own. The worker who selects a particular child and showers him with gifts, special privileges, or constant attention is promising a parental relationship he will be unable to sustain. Not only do other children and staff resent such favoritism, but sometimes the child will avoid the adult to avoid being labeled as somebody's "pet." We do not wish, however, to leave the impression that the disinterested and aloof worker is better performing his duties than the "overinvolved" one; it is better to offer a child too much than to offer him nothing.

Minimizing Adult Aversiveness

Disengaging from Hostile Encounters. It is remarkable how one child can take a composed and sensible adult, and in a short period of time transform this adult into an angry, confused and befuddled individual. This happens because the adult has learned to expect reasonable treatment from those he treats in a reasonable manner, but such a child does not operate like this. What starts out as a well-intentioned encounter often ends up as a violent power struggle or as two angry persons isolating themselves from one another.

Many disturbed and delinquent youth have learned to associate adults with negative situations. It seems appropriate for the child-care worker to make an effort to counter this tendency of the child to perceive adults negatively by, insofar as possible, minimizing negative interactions with the children. Thus, while strong punishment may surpress a specific behavior, it often has the unfortunate side effect of inhibiting social responsiveness or causing the child to withdraw from interaction with the punisher (Azrin and Holz, 1966). Yet, since many of these youngsters engage in very deviant behavior, it is easy for the adult to counter with harsh control techniques. And, no matter how benign an adult might attempt to be, the child's past experiences bias his perception of the present adult. It therefore takes considerable effort on the part of the adult to avoid becoming just another aversive person to the child. Some of the things the child-care worker might do to minimize his aversiveness to the child are discussed below.

The Power Struggle. Adlerian psychologists (e.g., Dreikurs, 1964) have described the tendency for some children to become locked in combat with an adult, with each party seeking to gain the upper hand. This situation is very common in residential treatment, and it is noted that some workers manage to get themselves entangled in such encounters more frequently than others. The model of such an exchange is well known to every parent: "I ain't! Yes you are, and this instant! No, I'm not, and you can't make me! Oh, yes, I can!" etc. Little incidents improperly handled have a way of escalating into something well beyond the proportion of the original act. While there are some struggles in which it is necessary that the adult carry through to "victory," there are just many situations where it would be better for all concerned if the adult could disengage from such an encounter. Such is illustrated by this account of a teacher in a power struggle with a 10-year-old disturbed boy:

> Billy had a way of getting me caught up in big fights over nothing. I really didn't realize how bad it had become until one day I ended up spanking him for refusing to blow his nose.

Such incidents occur when we "take up the challenge" that is thrown before us by a child. Some workers seem to be able to see a power struggle coming on and avoid it, while others more blindly walk right into such confrontations.

There are five phrases that are frequently heard as a power struggle shifts into gear; it may do the worker well to memorize these and think twice before he responds to the child who says them:

1. "I ain't gonna!"
2. "Forget you, man!"
3. "I don't care what you say!"
4. "You can't make me!"
5. "I'll do what I feel like!"

This list is certainly not all inclusive, and the worker will discover other remarks that likewise elicit from him a retort which serves only to escalate the warfare rather than redirect the child or resolve the issue. What happens is that both parties get themselves into a position where to capitulate would mean to lose face. The cardinal rule is to avoid putting youngsters or yourself in such situations if at all possible. Failing this, the worker must decide whether it is worth continuing this battle of personalities; if the issue is miniscule he will do best to disentangle himself from the controversy.

It has been stated that one of the attributes of the effective child-care worker is the ability to say no, mean no, and yet be able to save face if the child does not comply. While this should not be misinterpreted to mean that there is value *per se* in adults knuckling under in the face of childhood resistance, the point is that there are times when it is better to disengage from rather than pursue a deteriorating interaction. One of the better ways of doing this is to become silent or even walk away from the youngster; this is not equivalent to the admission of defeat, since the child is left wondering what the adult is planning to do. Another useful ploy is to delay action, perhaps with a comment like, "Well, there's no sense in arguing. That's the way it is. If you don't understand, we'll have to settle it later."

Sometimes it is best to let the child have the last say. Some youngsters have such "pride" that it is virtually impossible for them to yield to the adult officially. One gets the impression that they would be "spitting all the way to the electric chair" if they were pushed to that point. Therefore, if the child gives a semblance of compliance, it may be best for a while to ignore certain other gestures of defiance. For example, when a child is sent to his room for misbehaving, he may loudly slam the door on the way in. It will not usually be wise for the adult to respond to this challenge, e.g., bolting through the door with a new chastisement for the act of defiance, since he is in effect saying, "You can make me do it, but you can't control everything I do."

The Contaminated Situation. Let us assume that something has gone wrong in the interaction between worker and child; perhaps the adult has disappointed the child, perhaps the child has been restricted or punished in some way. In any case, the adult has temporarily acquired negative characteristics in the child's perception. Redl (1957) says of such a situation that the adult is, in effect, "contaminated." Normal interactions are now disrupted, and the child may be less responsive to the adult's influence attempts. While time itself may remedy most of these situations, the worker may wish to accelerate the return to normal interaction. This "decontamination" can be accelerated in a number of ways.

Frequently, communication is disrupted and the child resists the adults attempts to converse. It may be best to leave the child alone for a while and then return a little later with a neutral or positive comment (e.g., "It's almost time for supper, are you ready?"), hoping that the youngster will accept this bid for renewed interaction. The worker can also talk to the child in a monologue, not expecting the child to answer, but from time to time giving him a chance to reopen communication. Sometimes if the adult re-explains the situation that led to the problem, avoiding a condemning tone, the child will be willing to "forget" whatever it was that led to the difficulty. In any case, the adult should expect rebuff or sometimes hostile remarks from the child, and not be angered if his initial attempts fail.

Punishments or restrictions sometimes have a way of leaving hard feelings between the worker and child. Therefore, it is sometimes helpful if the adult can "decontaminate" himself after a restriction has been administered. For example, note the following account:

> Billy was sent to his room for fighting, and in about ten minutes I went to see if he was ready to come out. I used to say, "Time's up, you can come out now" to him, but this would mean that he would be angry or sulking for some time afterward. Today I said, "We want you to join us if you think you are ready to come back now." He said he wasn't mad any more and rejoined the group in good spirits.

This account suggests that it may be valuable to re-establish positive interactions when they have been disrupted by punishments or crisis in order to lessen the carryover of the negative aspects of the punishment to later situations. The principle of maintaining communication after a time of crisis applies to international conflict as well as to interpersonal conflict (McNeil, 1965).

Removing the Trust Barrier. One reason that adults are aversive to some youngsters is that the adult cannot be trusted. Trust is related to the child's perceptions of what adult intentions are. Many maladjusted children perceive adults as intending to deceive or exploit them. If the "trust barrier" is to be removed, the child must learn that adults are concerned with his welfare rather than with deceiving or exploiting him (Deutsch, 1962). This distrust is why it is so important that the adult always be honest in his dealings with children. It is important that the worker never deliberately lie to a youngster; it takes only one isolated instance where a child discovers the adult has lied to counter hundreds of times that the adult has attempted to establish his credibility.

From time to time, every worker makes a mistaken judgment that affects a particular child. In such a situation it will usually be best if the adult is able to face the child and admit his mistake. While some workers find this very difficult to do, the fact remains that the youngsters are usually aware of the adult's mistake anyway; any attempt to "cover up" will only cause the adult to be regarded with greater suspicion. We do not suggest that the adult should reveal his sundry errors in and out of the living situation; but in those matters directly effecting the child, credibility is of paramount importance. Mowrer (1966) has suggested that such an approach provides the client (here the child) the opportunity to learn appropriate behavior, such as honesty, by modeling the therapist's behavior.

The trust barrier must be eliminated gradually over a period of time. The worker will deserve the resistance he encounters if he is too obvious in his attempt to gain the child's "trust" (which sometimes means the worker wants the child to reveal the exciting things that lie dormant in the child's case history). A more subtle approach that respects the child's inability to trust the adult will likely produce better results:

> The supervisor was trying to find out what caused the big fight between the boys tonight, and was questioning Larry. Larry said, "I ain't talking. I don't trust you or anybody else around here!" The supervisor told him, "It's all right if you don't trust me. I probably wouldn't if I were in your place either. You haven't known me very long, and I can't think of one reason you should trust me." Larry obviously hadn't expected this answer, and after a pause said, "Well, at least you never lied to me . . . I don't think." He then proceeded to explain how the group fight came about.

Trust is a two-way arrangement. If the worker shows trust in the child, the child will be more inclined to trust the worker. But by way of warning it is unwise to expose a child to responsibilities he is unequipped to handle; as Redl (1966) suggests, we do not leave purses full of money lying around just to prove to the child that we trust him. Rather, we should "program" trust in small doses. Limited responsibilities appropriately assigned to a youngster will convey to him our trust but avoid the likelihood that he will violate that trust.

Certain institutional settings and management policies contribute to the maintenance of trust barriers. If searching a child's room for dangerous objects of contraband is necessary, and the youngsters are not receptive to the search, then the confirmation of distrust has been provided. While it is not possible to establish standards of privacy and search that will be appropriate to every setting, the fact remains that the more distrust that adults display in their dealings with the children, the more distrustful the youngsters will be. Such a situation was handled by one worker in the following manner:

> We knew from things the boys had said that Ronny had been in charge of hiding the stolen money. Ron was confronted. He first denied it and then challenged us to "go ahead and search if you want; you won't find anything." We told him that we wanted to trust the boys, and if we went snooping around in their stuff, it wouldn't show that we trusted them very much. But we knew that he had hidden the money somewhere, and since we were fair to him by not searching his stuff, he should be honest with us, too. He said he would have to talk with the other guys before he could tell us; he had a conference with the others and in a few minutes returned with the money.

The temptation to search the youngsters in such a situation is strong. Yet if the youth possesses any real delinquent skills, the adult is not apt to find the contraband anyway; a search will only contribute to the atmosphere of distrust. It must be conveyed that adults are not against youngsters in "cops-and-robbers" fashion, but that everyone gets along best if honesty prevails.

Capitalizing on Crisis. Even the youth who ordinarily has nothing to do with adults will be more receptive to them in certain crisis situations. A youngster who has consistently avoided adults may suddenly seek them out when he is hurt, sick, frightened, or lonely—seeming to abandon for the moment his well-entrenched defenses against adults. The growing body of research on the significance of crisis suggests that individuals may be much more susceptible to a helping relationship and much more responsive to therapeutic attempts at these times of stress (Caplan, 1961). Child-care workers have noted that their relationship with a particular youngster underwent a marked change after some crucial incident. Sometimes this is a case where the adult has been involved in handling a serious behavior problem, such as "running away." At other times the adult has provided support to the child when he did not know where to turn for help or was unable to ask for help. Such a situation is exemplified in the following account of a sudden shift in the valence of the relationship between a child-care worker and a 12-year-old boy:

> Before yesterday, Wayne avoided me like the plague. But, two nights ago when I was making final rounds, I discovered him curled up on the floor with a blanket. I noted that his bed was wet so I went to get him some dry pajamas. I sent him into the bathroom to change, and while he was gone I put clean linen on his bed. When he returned he said, in a surprised tone, "You fixed my bed." I said good night and thought that was the end of that. But ever since then he has been very positive toward me, eagerly complies with any request I make, and is almost constantly seeking me out to ask questions, visit, or tell me the latest "jokes" he has heard.

Children are particularly vulnerable at times of crisis. If an adult is able to help a child through a trying situation, it is possible that the child will reformulate his perception of that adult. While this does not imply that it is good for adults to reinforce the dependency behavior in children constantly, it does seem that with the aloof and distrustful child so frequently encountered in residential settings, almost any sign of reliance upon adults is welcomed. There is even some recent evidence that among disturbed children, the presence of dependency behavior is positively related to therapeutic change (Spivack and Swift, 1966). The literature on life-space interviewing (Redl, 1966) and crisis intervention provides guidance on how one might best manage many crisis situations. We will consider related issues again in Chapter VII when we discuss "Understanding the Stages of a Typical Temper Tantrum."

References

AICHHORN, A. 1935. *Wayward youth*. New York: Viking Press.

AZRIN, N. H., and W. C. HOLZ. 1966. Punishment. In Werner K. Honig, (Ed.), *Operant behavior: areas of research and application.* New York: Appleton-Century-Crofts.

CAPLAN, G. (Ed.). 1961. *Prevention of mental disorders in children.* New York: Basic Books.

DEUTSCH, MORTON. 1964. Cooperation and trust: some theoretical notes. In W. G. Bennis *et al.* (Eds.), *Interpersonal dynamics.* Homewood, Ill.: Dorsey Press.

DREIKURS, R., and V. SOLTZ. 1964. *Children: the challenge.* Des Moines: Meredith Press.

ERIKSON, E. H. 1963. *Childhood and society.* New York: W. W. Norton.

GOLDSTEIN, D. P., K. HELLER, and L. B. SECHREST. 1966. *Psychotherapy and the psychology of behavior change.* New York: John Wiley.

HARLOW, HARRY H. 1960. The nature of love. In M. L. Haimowitz and N. Haimowitz (Eds.), *Human development.* New York: Thomas Y. Crowell.

HOFFER, W. 1949. Deceiving the deceiver. In K. R. Eissler (Ed.), *Searchlights on delinquency.* New York: International Universities Press.

HUNTER, E. 1954. *The blackboard jungle.* New York: Simon and Schuster.

KRECH, D., R. CRUTCHFIELD, and E. BALLACHEY. 1962. *Individual in society.* New York: McGraw-Hill.

KVARACEUS, W., and WALTER MILLER. 1959. *Delinquent behavior.* Washington, D.C.: National Educational Association.

MCDERMOTT, J. F., S. FRAIBERG, and S. HARRISON. 1966. Utilization of transference behavior in residential treatment of the child. Paper presented at the American Association of Residential Children's Centers, October 30.

MCNEIL, E. B. 1960. Two styles of expression: motoric and conceptual. In D. R. Miller and G. E. Swanson (Eds.), *Inner conflict and defense.* New York: Henry Holt.

———. 1965. *The nature of human conflict.* Englewood Cliffs, N.J.: Prentice-Hall.

MINUCHIN, S., PAMELA CHAMBERLAIN, and PAUL GRAUBARD. 1966. A project to teach learning skills to disturbed delinquent children. Paper presented at the American Orthopsychiatric Association, San Francisco.

MOWRER, O. HOBART. 1966. The behavior therapies with special reference to modeling and imitation. *American Journal of Psychotherapy,* 20: 439–461.

REDL, FRITZ. 1966. *When we deal with children.* New York: Free Press.

———, and DAVID WINEMAN. 1957. *The aggressive child.* Glencoe, Ill.: Free Press.

RUBIN, THEODORE. 1961. *Lisa and David.* New York: Macmillan.

SPIVACK, G., and M. S. SWIFT. 1966. The Devereux elementary school behavior rating scales: a study of the nature and organization of achievement related disturbed classroom behavior. *Journal of Special Education* (Fall, 1966), 1: 71–90.

SULLIVAN, HARRY S. 1953. *The interpersonal theory of psychiatry.* New York: W. W. Norton.

III
PROGRAM ACTIVITIES
Their Selection and Use in a Therapeutic Milieu

James K. Whittaker

The Place of Activities in the Therapeutic Milieu

> A boy, alone, sits on a fence staring sadly, a tear wending its way down his face, at a group of children playing in a yard. This is the lonely isolate, hurting inside to be able to join in but so threatened by relationships with himself and others that he cannot (DeNoon, 1965, p. 88).

All of us who have worked with disturbed children will recognize the plight of the "empty" child: the child who cannot make friends easily or who considers himself so "nothing" that nobody could want to be his friend. One of the most important components of any treatment plan for such a youngster would have to include his participation in carefully selected and supervised activity programs, where he could begin to learn new peer-relating skills and develop his own embryonic sense of self worth. Skilled clinicians have come to think of activity programs as not merely a pleasant adjunct to psychotherapy, but as a meaningful and necessary part of a child's treatment. Redl and Wineman speak of activity programs as a "full-fledged therapeutic tool"; they state quite emphatically that "Programming can play a specific role in the clinical task on its own, not only a 'time-filling' substitute for psychiatric contacts during the rest of the day" (Redl and Wineman, 1957, p. 393).

Some theorists have shown that activities have a reality and a behavior influencing power in their own right (Gump and Sutton-Smith, 1965, p. 414), while others have pointed out that some specific developmental needs of children are met through activities: mastery of skills, release of aggression, mastery of relationships and the art of sublimation (Konopka, 1954, pp. 141–146). Play, as described by Bettelheim, (1950, p. 218), is that area where the child tests and develops his independence and where he learns to hold his own with his peers. Obviously, such an important part of the child's world, "play" should not be looked upon as a uniform event or as a totally random activity. Piaget has given us some insight into the complex normative structure governing what at first glance appears to be unplanned activity (1951). Erikson gives us some insight into the potentialities of child's play as a medium for learning:

> Child's play is not the equivalent of adult play . . . it is not recreation. The adult steps sidewards into another reality; the playing child advances forward to new stages of mastery (Erikson, 1950, pp. 194–195).

Finally, Redl and others have noted the tremendous impact of the structure of games and activities on those participating in them (Redl, 1966, p. 87).

What, then are we speaking of when we discuss this rather complex subject of activity programming? For our purpose here, we may think of "program" as any activity in which children are engaged either with other children or with adults. Clearly, this rather loose definition of program encompasses many things, but it is well to remember that the child's world is a world of play. With or without the intervention of helping adults, activities have benefit both for the individual child and for the group. Perhaps no other medium is better designed to allow individual children to acquire a sense of competency and mastery over their environment. Activities also provide opportunities to practice group participation, to experiment with new roles in a small group situation, and to try out newly acquired peer-relating skills.

Activities may also be used as diagnostic tools to assess not only individual children, but also group structure and decision-making processes. Most of the case records accompanying children to residential treatment centers have a surplus of intrapsychic evaluative data, but a dearth of material pertaining to how the child functions in a group situation. We are often quite aware of a child's learning deficiencies, but tend to overlook the fact that many children simply do not know how to have fun. The mastery of program activities provides them with at least one concrete and marketable peer skill. Finally, if we truly believe that activity programs are not merely a pleasant addition to psychotherapy, but function as "full-fledged therapeutic tools," then activity programs must be a guaranteed commodity in the therapeutic milieu and not something held out solely as a reward for "good" behavior. This is not to suggest that we always present a wide range of activities to all children at all times. It would make little sense, for instance, to suggest a game of chess to a child wildly out of control. On the other hand, many of the presenting problems of the youngsters: poor peer relations, aggressive outbursts, and low self images can often be treated better in the context of an activity than a fifty-minute office interview. It is, therefore, important that we not limit the use of this "tool" to those times when children are in good psychological shape.

How To Select an Activity

"There's nothin' to do around this crummy place." Many child-care workers have been greeted by this cheery acclamation when they have arrived for duty on an afternoon shift. The process of selecting and carrying out a successful and beneficial activity program is complex and difficult. It involves evaluating such variables as skill and interests of the children, staff coverage, available materials, and the mood of the group. Other slightly more distant variables may be crucial to the success of a particular activity; this class of variable includes such things as weather, time of day, and other such "atmospheric variables." Nothing can ruin that carefully planned baseball game quicker than an unexpected cloudburst and pity the poor child-care worker who does not have an alternative program available when such an unforeseen event occurs.

Our purpose in this section of the paper will be to elucidate six activity-setting dimensions and three individual variables which will provide a framework for the selection and evaluation of activities. Hopefully, it will answer one of the questions most frequently asked by the child-care workers, "How do I know which activity to choose?"

The six activity-setting dimensions derive largely from the work of Dr. Robert Vinter at the University of Michigan School of Social Work (Vinter, 1967, pp. 95–110). Vinter's formulations were based on the earlier work of Gump and his associates.

Every child-care worker knows that he can do certain things even before the start of the activity that will influence the course the activity will follow. Group-work practitioners know that manipulation of space, time, props, and materials can alter the way in which groups will approach and carry out activities (Churchill, 1959); but the activities themselves, also have "built-in" dimensions, or component parts, which have a good deal to do with the behavior of the participants. Since these six dimensions are relevant to all activities, they bear obvious relevance to the child-care worker who is attempting to select an activity for his group. The six dimensions are explained below (Vinter, 1967, pp. 98–100):

1. *Prescriptiveness of the pattern of constituent performances.* This is simply the degree and range of rules required by the activity. For example, contrast the complex set of rules governing a game of chess and the relatively few rules governing a simple children's game like "Leapfrog." "Monopoly" is a more prescriptive board game than "Chutes and Ladders," and arts and crafts activities usually have a fairly high degree of rules and structure compared to an activity like free swimming, which has a low degree of prescriptiveness.
2. *Institutionalized controls governing participant activity.*

This refers to the form and source of controls exercised over participants during the activity. Controls are sometimes embodied in a person (participant) or in a person representing a body of rules (umpire, referee) or simply in a set of rules commonly accepted by the participants. Controls, whether personal or impersonal, not only determine the conduct of the activity at a given moment but also determine who may participate. The "It" person in a children's game may exercise a high degree of control over fellow participants (as in "Redlight" or "Simon Says"), or a relatively low degree of control (as in "Hide and Seek").

3. *Provision for physical movement.* This is the extent to which participants are required or permitted to move about in the activity setting. Some activities (running, swimming) have considerably more provision for physical movement than others (contract bridge).
4. *Competence required for performance.* This dimension refers to the minimum level of ability required to participate in the activity, but not to the competence required to excel or win. For example, some activities require a low level of beginning competence for participation (group singing, dodge ball) while others require a fairly well developed skill (water skiing, horse-back riding).
5. *Provision for participant interactiveness.* This is the way in which the activity-setting locates and engages participants so that interaction among them is required or provoked. For example, building individual airplane models in a crafts' room would have less provision for participant interactiveness than a game of baseball or "tug-o-war." Interaction may be verbal and/or nonverbal.
6. *Reward structure.* This refers to the types of rewards available, their abundance or scarcity, and the manner in which they are distributed. Some rewards are intrinsic to the activity (creating a piece of sculpture), while others derive from secondary sources in the setting (receiving praise for excelling, releasing tension legitimately, and improving skill). The distribution of rewards may be distinguished from their scarcity or abundance, although these characteristics are related. Obviously, if there are fewer rewards than

participants, they must be unequally distributed. In competitive play—whatever intrinsic gratifications are derived by all players through participation—only one side may win. In many activities, certain positions or roles provide more rewards for their occupants than do others. In baseball, for example, the pitcher, catcher, and infield may gain greater rewards than their fellow players in the outfield.

The above six activity-setting dimensions represent a condensation of Vinter's lucid and complete explanation of the six dimensions. Deletions, additions, and paraphrasing were used where necessary because of the limited scope of this chapter. For a more complete explanation of the dimensions, the reader is referred to the Activity Paper (Vintner, 1967).

One final dynamic in examining the reward structure concerns *who* is leading the activity. For example, some activities become almost completely associated with a particular staff member to the point where suggestion of the activity on the part of another staff member will lead to apathetic responses or significantly less enjoyment on the part of the participants.

Individual Variables

Having then looked at some criteria for assessing activities, we may turn to a discussion of individual and group variables to be considered when choosing an activity:

1. *Skill.* Skill here refers to the level of the child's competency in participating in activities and would include such things as physical dexterity and motor coordination, as well as specific athletic, mechanical, or crafts skills. Many children come to us with relatively few specific skills, though their interest might be keen in specific areas. Basically, a question focused on this variable asks, "What is this child capable of doing right now?"

2. *Motivation.* This refers to the child's willingness to participate in activities and obviously has a lot to do with the child's relationship with the child-care worker. It has many ramifications for the process of selecting an activity. For ex-

ample, the more complex and difficult the activity, the higher the child's motivation will have to be in order to insure its successful completion. Conversely, children with relatively low motivation to join in activities may be lured into participation with activities whose rewards are both immediate and abundant.

3. *On tap control.* This refers to the amount of self control available to the child at a given time. One would not recommend a game of chess for a hyperactive child who has been struggling to control his behavior in school all day. With hyperactive aggressive children, we do not always wait for a child to be completely in control before attempting to engage him in an activity. Rather, we may engage him in an activity for the purpose of controlling his behavior.

Group Variables

In planning program one must keep in mind certain group phenomena that may influence the course of the activity. Some of the more important of these are group solidarity (cohesion), group composition, and groop mood. If we are working with a loosely assembled group where there is little cohesion esprit and solidarity, we might better think in terms of parallel activities, rather than those that require a good deal of interaction and interdependence among the members (e.g., model building rather than soccer). As for group composition, obviously, the more heterogeneous the grouping, the more difficult it will be to find an activity all members can participate in and enjoy. Finally, the child-care worker must use his own sensitivities to assess the mood of the group: a spontaneous suggestion of an unplanned hike may be just the thing for the group of latency-age youngsters who have been using massive amounts of control completing a project in school and seem ready to "bust out."

In summation, the child-care worker does not go through all of the activity-setting dimensions, individual variables, and group variables every time he plans a program. To do this as an exercise may be useful (Vinter has analyzed two divergent activities, swimming and arts and crafts, in the program paper); but to try and control for all of the aforementioned variables before we made a program decision would be disastrous. Rather, we would use the dimensions and the individual and group variables to plan for particularly difficult activity times; finally, we may use them as guidelines to dissect and analyze our particular successes as well as our utter disasters (see Appendix I).

When to Use an Activity

The maintenance of the rather delicate balance between individual and group psychotherapy, remedial education and program activities is one of the most crucial issues in any good therapeutic residence. Probing the depths of a child's psyche, helping him to overcome a learning problem, or teaching him an alternative behavior are all laudable goals, but the milieu must provide some respite from the rigors and pains of psychic change. This is not to suggest for a moment that skillful use of activities need be completely isolated from the individual treatment modality and, indeed, it can often serve to enhance it. For many youngsters activities may constitute the key medium in which growth and development is enhanced. Thus, our view of activities is that they constitute what amounts to a "full-fledged therapeutic tool," which can be immensely useful in managing behavior as well as in initiating and fomenting real therapeutic progress.

Transition Time Activities

One of the key problems faced by all child-care workers is that of moving children through the routines and activities of the day. Children must arise in the morning, go off to school, come to lunch and supper, prepare for bedtime and group activities. Indeed, much of the child's day is spent moving toward or away from the routines of the milieu. If the child-care worker depends solely upon his "authority" to move children through the structures of the day, he soon finds himself making "issues" over fairly simple rules and getting into power struggles where the only goal of the child seems to be, "Whatever you tell me to do, I'm going to do the opposite!" If, on the other hand, the counselor resorts solely to direct appeals, he soon finds himself laying his relationship on the line for every demand and request. Direct appeal also presupposes that the child is motivated to follow the routine (go to school, come to lunch, etc.), an assumption I doubt that many child-care workers would care to make all of the time.

Thus, we have found it useful to add activities to our bag of management tools. These activities are by definition short term, since they end as soon as the child is engaged in the routine. Their primary purpose is diversion and, if possible, their focus should be on the counselor as the "central figure." Thus, games like "Follow the Leader" or "Redlight" have been found to be quite useful in guiding the children from the school room to the lunch table. It helps if certain games become associated with certain times of the day, as the child sees the game as a "marker" which indicates the proximity of the particular routine. One counselor made very successful use of a "timing game" with a child who had particular difficulties getting dressed in the morning (see Chapter IV, p. 124).

Waiting for an activity or a routine to begin can often be the source of a great deal of frustration for the impulsive youngster. One therapeutic camp keeps a long rope outside of the dining hall to be used for group high-jumping if the dinner bell is late. One need not think of elaborate materials for these activities and, indeed, the contents of one's own pockets often provides ample props for successful short-term programs. Thus, the stopwatch may be used to "See how fast you can run to school"; the penny becomes the object of some sleight of hand, or the counter in a game of penny-pitch. The fascination with a few simple card tricks may be enough to keep the group occupied until the broken projector gets fixed. Finally, since these activities are by nature short term, the counselor might wish to use a whole sequence of them while skillfully moving the youngsters from one part of the program to another.

Individual and Group Activities

Activities may be structured around the needs of a particular child or may be designed for the hygiene of the entire group. A newcomer to the group might have a particular skill or interest that could serve as his inroad to the group if included in a carefully prepared activity by the child-care worker. Generally speaking, it is well to think of activities that tax the control of the individual child only slightly at first; here, we substitute the depersonalized control of the activity for the internal control which the child is lacking. For example, the counselor might wish to outline the rules for "dodge-ball," rather than leave each dispute to be arbitrated by the children.

The whole question of when to use program activities carries with it a certain aversion to the whole notion of programming. No one likes to think of himself as being "programmed" and the thought of a rigidly designed activity structure (swimming at 2:00, then arts and crafts at 3:00) does not fit with the creative abilities of the child-care worker, much less with the needs of the impulsive child. The goal should be one of weaving activities into the fabric of the milieu, taking into account the needs, interests, and limitations of the children as well as the abilities of the counselor and the resources available to him.

One way to approach the problem is the use of programming through the project method. Here the counselor starts with the kernel of an idea from a child, or group of children and builds it into an activity or series of activities that may carry on for days and provide many levels of rewards for the participants. The following group log may help to explain one such program.

Today Bobby greeted me and told me that the class had just concluded the unit on American Indians. He expressed some interest in making a bow and arrow, but said, "It probably wouldn't work anyway." I approached Vince and Rick on the idea and they seemed to be enthusiastic. The four of us set about gathering sticks for the arrows and discovered a natural "teepee" in some large bushes. Two boys began at once to clear the area while Bobby began work on his bow and arrow. By now, Carol [counselor] had become involved and began making Indian bracelets and trinkets out of scraps of leather. I spoke with Linda [teacher] after school and she said she would introduce the idea of an Indian exhibit in school . . . (C.L., 9/21/63).

This project, which began with one boy's idea to make a bow and arrow, culminated in an Indian day about a week later, complete with ceremonial dancing, totempole making, and a cookout. Within the general framework of the program, there was tremendous room for individual tastes and skills. Thus, one child spent most of his time painting shields, while another was engaged in the rather formidable task of "guarding the campsite."

In short, the richest source of inspiration for program comes from the children themselves and it is the task of the child-care worker to refine, modify and build upon the idea of the child.

Suggestions

This final section deals with helpful program hints culled from the collective experience of many child-care workers. They reflect, I believe, what is the goal of every child-care worker in a therapeutic residence: to relate the world of fun and activities to the child whose ability to enjoy success is often overshadowed by his fear that "I can't do anything right."

1. One of the key tools of the child-care worker in executing a successful activity is the use of his own enthusiasm. The counselor who is actively involved in the game (and who is quite obviously enjoying himself) provides a model for the child of how a person relates to an activity. It is no small task, however, to juggle the roles of "helping adult" and "playmate," and counselors should guard against becoming

so involved in the activity that they cannot step out from time to time to manage a crisis.

2. Activities should be ended when they are going well and while the children are enjoying themselves. Many counselors have experienced dismay when the activity they have been running all evening crumbles before their eyes when it is left to run out. It is better to leave the child with a positive picture of the activity at its high point, rather than with a negative picture of its demise.

3. The timing and sequence of activities are important variables to control. For example, large group activities first thing in the morning are not usually successful because the individual egos of the youngsters are too fragmented and shaky to be exposed to mass group games. Similarly, body contact sports right before bedtime are likely to contage the group into erotic and aggressive play at a time when children are undressing and taking showers. (Here let us explode for all time the myth that "a few laps around the track" or a "wrestling match" will "tire them out and make them ready for sleep.")

4. Often the counselor must rejuvenate and alter old activities to make them more attractive to the youngsters. One counselor changed the old and familiar game of "ghosts" to "rocketships" and enjoyed a good deal of success with it. We must also make allowance for the child's inability to delay gratification; thus a rapid rotation of hitters may be better than a conventional game of baseball.

5. With ego-damaged children whose skill level is often pitifully low, we must be careful not to place too much emphasis on the "finished product." Similarly, the counselor should use his own skills to complement those of the child and not be overly concerned over "who did what."

6. Despite the most careful planning of an activity, the counselor may be faced with the situation of seeing it turn to dust before his eyes as a result of the pathology of the individual youngster or the mood of the group. He must be ever ready to switch activities in midstream as the need arises.

7. Many child-care workers ask the question, "How do I start an activity?" The answer simply is do it! It is quite easy

to fall into the trap of wanting to "get the whole group together" (and quiet) before beginning, when often it is the lure of the activity itself that will do most to interest the youngsters.

8. Generally speaking, when working with a younger group, it is better to begin with parallel activities, i.e., those which do not require interaction between the members. Thus, it is better to have six individual model ships and not one giant aircraft carrier for "everyone to work on." Participation and facilitative interaction are goals to be sought, but later as the group develops.

9. Similarly, when beginning to work with a younger group, it is wise for the child-care worker to reserve the greater portion of decision-making for himself. This alleviates somewhat the problem of each child having to negotiate with every other child what the activity is to be.

10. Finally, the child-care worker should not attempt those activities in which he is not skilled or does not feel comfortable, just because he or she feels some need to be the "compleat counselor." It would be far better for him to develop those skills and interests which are most important to him, for there is usually a wide enough variation among child-care staffs that the children are exposed to a whole range of different activities.

Appendix I

The "goodness of fit" between any theoretical model and its "real-life" counterpart is at best a tentative union. With this in mind, the application of the Vinter material along with the individual variables should represent to the child-care worker a somewhat incomplete framework designed to help him answer the question, "How do I select an activity?" I suspect there will be some disagreement as to the "ratings" assigned to the different activities, as well as to the eight representations of the program participants. This is as it should be, for I believe all of us are agreed that neither activities nor children may be divided into neatly defined categories. If, however, the following exercise in some way provides a rudimentary framework for the analysis of activities and the people who participate in them, our purpose will have been well served.

The following eight "program types" represent all of the possible combinations when one controls for the variables of *Skill, Motivation,* and *Control:*

PROGRAM TYPE	SKILL	MOTIVATION	CONTROL
A	High	High	High
B	High	High	Low
C	High	Low	Low
D	Low	Low	Low
E	Low	Low	High
F	Low	High	High
G	Low	High	Low
H	High	Low	High

The following behavioral descriptions will help to illustrate:

Type A

This child has high skill, motivation, and control; he is able to participate in a wide range of individual and group activities. He can perform demanding tasks for moderate reward and is able to postpone gratification. This youngster probably "programs" quite well for himself.

Type B

Highly skilled and motivated, this child is plagued by a poor control structure; any activity for him must substitute external controls for his own lack of internal control. He is easily contaged by others—thus it would be well to avoid mass group activities, but he can certainly function well in small group situations.

Type C

This child has an abundance of natural ability, but is unable (or unwilling) to utilize it effectively; rewards for him should be abundant and immediate. Controls must be provided externally, but the fewer rules the better. This child will probably work best in a one to one situation.

Type D

This youngster presents a real challenge: he is poorly motivated, relatively "empty" of skills and has extremely poor control over his own impulses. We should begin with very simple activities that will assure almost "instant success"; in addition, we must provide a good deal of external support to supplement his poorly integrated control structure. Finally, we should provide a good deal of space for physical movement and not expect that this child will stick to any one thing for a very long period of time.

Type E

This child is poorly motivated and unskilled, but presents no great control problem. He is probably a shy, withdrawing youngster who feels rebuffed by his peers and has a very low self image. He too needs immediate successes and uncomplicated games and projects. Lots of help and praise will enhance his development, and the rest of the group could help in this respect.

Type F

This child has good motivation and control, but a low skill level. He is a clumsy youngster, who does poorly at athletics and group games. He is willing and able to work on mastery experiences and could probably use some sort of a plan for skill development so that his ego will not be crushed every time he misses the basket or strikes out.

Type G

This child has low skill, a faulty control structure, but really wants to "do well." We must begin with activities that require a low beginning degree of competence and have plenty of provision for physical movement. Probably our most difficult task with this particular child will be getting him to accept the fact that skill or control take time to develop and that he should not become discouraged in the process.

Type H

This youngster has good ability and control, but is poorly motivated to participate in activities. We think immediately of the sociologically trained delinquent who stands aloof from the "fun and games" of the residence. The key here is, of course, relationship development and finding the most meaningful reward that will enhance his entry into the group (peer status, friendship, privileges).

Next by matching each participant type with the activity dimensions we arrive at an ideal activity profile for each of the types (see the Ideal Activity Profile on pp. 116–117).

Thus, Type E (poorly skilled and motivated, but presenting no great control problem) would require an activity that had a low degree of prescriptiveness, but provided a goodly amount of external control. In addition, the rewards would have to be fairly abundant, but the competency needed to attain them would have to be minimal. Hence, we might try finger painting or papier-mâché with him, but definitely

Ideal Activity Profile

Participant Types	Prescriptiveness	Control	Prov. Phys.
A	High	Low–High	Low
B	Medium	High	High
C	Low	High	High
D	Low	Low	High
E	Low	High	Medium
F	High	High	Medium
G	Low	Low	High
H	High	High	Low

Common Activity Scale

Activity	Prescriptiveness	Controls	Physical Movement
Swimming	Low	Low	High
Model Building	High	High	Low
Clay Molding	Low	Low	Low
Fingerpainting	Low	Low	Medium
Papier-Mâché	Low	Medium	Low
Origami	High	High	Low
Copper Enameling	Medium	High	Low
Lanyard Making	Medium	Medium	Low
Baseball	High	High	Medium–High
Touch Football	Medium	Medium	High
Hockey	Medium	High	High
Kick Ball	Low–Medium	Medium	Medium
Dodge Ball	Low	Low	High
Red Rover	Medium	Medium	High
Tag	Low	Low	High
Chinese Tag	Medium	Medium	Medium–High
Redlight	High	High	Medium
Simon Says	High	High	Medium
Hide 'n' Seek	Low	Medium	Medium
Checkers	High	High	Low
Chess	High	High	Low
Monopoly	High	High	Low
Chutes 'n' Ladders	Medium	Medium	Medium

Ideal Activity Profile

Participant Types	Reward	Competency	Part. Inter
A	Medium	High	High
B	Medium	High	Medium–Low
C	High	High	Low
D	High	Low	Low
E	High	Low	Medium
F	Medium	Low	High
G	Medium	Low	Low
H	High	High	High

Common Activity Scale

Activity	Reward	Competence	Part. Interact.
Swimming	High	Low	Low
Model Building	High	High	Low
Clay Modeling	High	Low	Low
Fingerpainting	High	Low	Low
Papier-Mâché	High	Low	Low
Origami	High	High	Low
Copper Enameling	High	Medium	Low
Lanyard Making	High	Low	Low
Baseball	Medium	High	High
Touch Football	High	Medium	High
Hockey	Medium	High	High
Kick Ball	Medium	Medium	Medium
Dodge Ball	High	Low	High
Red Rover	Medium	Low	High
Tag	High	Low	High
Chinese Tag	High	Medium–High	High
Redlight	Medium	Low	Low
Simon Says	Medium	High	Medium–Low
Hide 'n' Seek	High–Medium	Low	Low
Checkers	Medium	Medium	Medium
Chess	High	High	High
Monopoly	Medium–High	High	High
Chutes 'n' Ladders	Medium	Medium	Medium

not origami or copper enameling. In either case, we would do well to substitute for the lack of internal control by keeping the group small and the counselor close to the child. If thinking of outdoor games, we might try tag or dodge-ball, but would not be wise to think of Chinese tag or baseball, as they would require a higher level of beginning competence.

Finally, twenty-three common activities were rated on the Vinter scale; it is now possible to link up each activity with the participants who can successfully use it. Thus, Monopoly becomes a good activity for types A and H and possibly C, but is certainly not a good choice for types D and E (see the Common Activity Scale on pp. 116–117).

References

BETTELHEIM, BRUNO. 1950. *Love is not enough*. Glencoe, Ill.: Free Press.

CHURCHILL, SALLY. 1959. Prestructuring group content. *Social Work*, 4(3): 52–59.

DENOON, BARBARA. 1965. Horses, bait and chocolate cake. In Henry W. Maier (Ed.), *Group work as part of residential treatment*. New York: National Association of Social Work.

ERIKSON, ERIK H. 1950. *Childhood and society*. New York: W. W. Norton.

GUMP, PAUL, and BRIAN SUTTON-SMITH. 1965. "Therapeutic Play Techniques." In Nicholas J. Long, William C. Morse and Ruth G. Newman (Eds.), *Conflict in the classroom*. Belmont, Calif.: Wadsworth.

KONOPKA, GISELA. 1954. *Group work in the institution*. New York: Association Press.

PIAGET, JEAN. 1950. *Play, dreams and imitation in childhood*. New York: W. W. Norton.

REDL, FRITZ. 1966. *When we deal with children*. New York: Free Press.

———, and DAVID WINEMAN. 1957. *The aggressive child.* Glencoe, Ill.: Free Press.

VINTER, ROBERT D. 1967. Program activities: an analysis of their effects on participant behavior. In Robert D. Vinter (Ed.), *Group work practice.* Ann Arbor, Mich.: Campus Publishers.

IV
MANAGING WAKE-UP BEHAVIOR

James K. Whittaker

Each day most adults awake at a regular time, get out of bed, clean up, eat breakfast, and start their daily activities. So regular and automatic does this process become that we scarcely give it a second thought. If our alarm clock failed to work, we would probably awaken on schedule; if we did not feel particularly alert or had had a restless night, we would still be able to muddle through the demands of the morning on schedule. By way of contrast, many of the disturbed children we work with in residential settings find morning a difficult task to manage; waking up, getting out of bed, dressing, getting to breakfast, and getting off to school may be major hurdles for the child to overcome. By the time he finally arrives at school, he may have been involved in several fights with peers and a protracted argument with an adult. It is not difficult for us to imagine how the remainder of his day may be hampered by this poor beginning.

Perhaps the primary reason so many of our children experience difficulty in the morning is that during this time they are least able to deal with the other people, tasks, and objects

This chapter was prepared with the help of Margaret Komives, formerly a child-care worker at the Walker Home.

that are part of the milieu. During the wake-up period, the children progress from a primary investment in body awareness, inner thoughts, dream remnants, and encapsulation from the outside world to a direct confrontation with the tasks of dressing, eating breakfast, and moving off to school. Stated simply, they must cease turning inward and begin to deal with the outside world again.

Waking Up

After ten hours of sleep, isolation, and uninvolvement, a child finds it difficult to manage the task of beginning a new day. Typically, waking up may signify reengagement with a counselor who was forced to restrain a child physically the night before; similarly it may mean a new confrontation with an angry roommate who is out to "get him." Waking up signals an end to the warm security of the child's bed and an entrance into the cold and much less manageable world of the milieu. Needless to say, the child-care worker's actions at this stage are crucial, for these children almost invariably wake up with at least one foot on the wrong side of the bed.

During this initial stage, the counselor should move slowly and quietly around the children and speak in moderate tones to allow for the different waking-up and tuning-in rate of each child. Some children may awaken in surly moods after a disturbing dream and may be "moving at full speed" by the time we arrive. The question of whether to deal with the dream material during this early wake-up period is a complex one. Bettelheim (1950) has dealt with this particular issue in detail. Other children tend to wake up gradually, turn over and go back to sleep and then finally awaken. It is advisable at these times for the counselor to insist quietly upon the rules that are built into the morning routine: don't disturb other children, remain in your own room until dressed, and talk in modulated tones. The counselor moves from room to room attempting to help the child meet the new day by communicating with him on both a verbal and a nonverbal level. This may mean a comment about the weather prediction for the day, a comment about what kind of clothes are needed for a day like this, or a comment about what the counselor sees as he looks out of the window of the child's room. The conversation might take the form of some comment or question about something a child has accomplished the previous evening, but this is not the time to recall the huge upset or the disturbing phone call to home. The conversation should be chatty and informative rather than deep and psychologically probing. It should be concerned with the realities of the room, the other children, the routine for the day, and the day's activity. One result of the quiet conversational approach is that the child will be focused on the child-care worker. This direct focus on the worker and the reaffirmation of his interest in the child will tend to add leverage to his management actions later in the morning routine when he wants to reduce the interaction and contagion between children who are dressing. The children can gradually become engaged with each other through actions, low-keyed directions, and conversation.

Engaging a child nonverbally to demonstrate continuing interest in him is a good early-morning approach. For example, this might mean pulling up his shade, putting away some clean articles of clothing, putting his underwear on his bed, or picking up a toy and putting it on his shelf. The key to helping a child through his first task of waking up seems to be to avoid rushing or pushing children, saving exuberance for later in the day. This should be a time for quiet activity and dependence on the routine of the morning to carry the child through until he is better able to use his own resources to cope with the demands of the milieu. Some children will be able to accomplish this much more quickly than others. For most of the children, however, the process of waking up is a slow one. In a sense, each child has developed his own rate for reentering the milieu and if, for some reason, the child-care worker decides to accelerate or retard this rate, management difficulties may occur (Redl and Wineman, 1957, pp. 292–294). For example, Bettelheim (1950, esp. pp. 83–115) has noted that many disturbed children spend their first waking minutes in a slow ritualistic examination of body parts, almost as if they are checking to see if they are the same person who went to sleep the night before. A certain amount of this self examination must be tolerated during the early wake-up period. If the child-care worker tries to urge the child too rapidly or if he interprets this behavior to the child as simply a "stalling technique," he is likely to encounter management difficulties with the child later in the morning route. Two examples may help to explain more fully.

John, the counselor, was encountering particular difficulties in early mornings with his group of adolescent boys. A naturally exuberant and outgoing person, he would engulf the boys each morning with wave upon wave of enthusiasm, usually related to a particular activity they were going to join in later that afternoon. This somewhat overly enthusiastic approach was usually met with one of two responses. Sometimes the group would resist partaking in the first routine of the day, breakfast, and would lie around on their beds, cursing John and saying they were "fed up" with him and they "weren't goin' to do nothin'." At other times he really would get them enthusiastic and they would begin running around the dormitory at a heightened pace, wanting to start the activity then and there.

Another counselor, Bill, had no such early morning difficulties with the group. His approach was simply to come in in the morning and go to the bed of the boy who happened to wake up first. He would then pull a deck of cards from his pocket and usually without any verbal communication begin to deal out a hand of "Tunk," a game with which the boys were all familiar and one they enjoyed playing. Then, later, as other boys awoke, they could choose either to participate in this game or to watch it so that, by the time everybody was awake, each boy was participating in the game in either an active or a passive fashion. There was little conversation and yet each boy's attention was focused on the game; and Bill was, of course, the central focus of the game. In this manner, by putting something between himself and the children—in this case, an activity with cards which they enjoyed—he was able, in a sense, to shape this wake-up period without moving in too fast or without getting overly involved.

Dressing Routines

The first major task confronting the child is getting dressed. The same body concerns that marked the period of undressing in the evening are also present in the morning, and this can be a period of much resistance from the children. There is also a good probability that behavioral contagion will be high at this time with boys seeing each other in various stages of dress and undress. However, if we have successfully engaged the child in looking forward to the events of the new day at all, our management actions now will be easier.

Children respond differently to the various aids we can offer at this point. Beginning with milder aids and moving to more substantial ones, here are a few suggestions. With some children, the breakfast incentive can be used. For example, the new cereals, the hot chocolate, or the English muffins will often help a child arise, get dressed, and go downstairs. Perhaps the possibility of a child preparing part of his own breakfast or cooking something for another child will be a sufficient incentive to get him dressed and downstairs into the kitchen. Some children respond rather quickly to the mention of cartoons on television, a downstairs activity that does not require much interaction with other children.

Often, the lure of an unfinished project from the arts and crafts room is enough to bring a boy downstairs and away from the bedroom area. For example, the model airplane might need a final coat of paint, or the picture could be finished in the dining room before school. These projects in the morning should be very short term and should not be so involved that the child cannot leave them to move either to breakfast or to school when the time arrives. One successful counselor had the foresight to keep a number of half-completed lanyards in her pocket for the children to work on even while they were walking to school.

This is not the ideal time of the day for total group activities because many children are simply not ready to deal with the group as a whole this early in the day. Simple games, however, can often be used to help motivate a child to get dressed. One game children respond to most positively at this time of day involves the counselor's timing the child to see how long it takes for him to put on a particular article of clothing.

For example, "I'll count and see how long it takes you to get your underwear on" is one game that might be used. Or, "Let's see. I'll bet that if I stand in the hall and count to twenty, you could beat me and get your underwear on by fifteen. Okay? You tell me when to start counting." Or sometimes a hint of a challenge might be enough to get the child started: "Well, if it took you 40 to put on your underwear, I bet you couldn't put on your shirt and dungarees in 25." The amount of time the counselor picks assures that the child will win. In each case, it is wise to break down the parts of the dressing routine and not say simply, "I'll time you to see how long it takes you to get dressed." The fact is, that once a child has his underwear and socks on, the motivation to complete the process and his involvement with the counselor are greater and carry him through to the end of the task. This may be broken down even further for the child who has greater difficulty in dressing to the count of ten for socks, five for pants, five for tee shirts The child progresses through the dressing routine and does not see it as an insurmountable problem.

There is a certain etiquette that counselors should follow during this period, particularly female counselors. It is wise to avoid entering the child's room. This insures privacy and allows the motivated child to "trick" the counselor by getting all his clothes on by the count of twenty. This is also a time when counselors are likely to walk in unwittingly on boys engaged in masturbatory activities. As Redl has noted (1966, pp. 380–381), it is wise at these times to bow out gracefully, as if one had walked in on any other kind of private activity. Attempts at moralizing or an over-emphasis on behavioral interpretation will only lead to a "hangover" effect later in the day. The only time one would probably intervene would be if this behavior was being imitated by other boys; then one could suggest that the boy engaging in the activity dress in another room by himself. Finally, much can be communicated by the attitude of the counselor helping the child to dress. Next to feeding a child, clothing him is one of the basic tasks of parents. It is also one of the least interesting jobs, and counselors have to guard against appearing aggravated or irritated that children cannot do more for themselves. This is a time when much can be done toward the task of building a relationship. For example:

Eddie appeared in camp as a cool and reserved delinqent. He had little conversation with any of the adults and remained pretty much to himself. On the fourth day at camp, he very calmly expressed a desire to one of his counselors that he would like to go home. When the counselor questioned him, he answered with a shrug of the shoulders and the statement: "Why should I want to stay in this baby place?"

Earlier in the week, Bill, the counselor, had noted that Eddie took a great deal of pride in dressing and spent a good portion of the morning getting ready. He had later noticed that Eddie's clothing supply was running low and that it was probably time to have some laundry done. Without commenting further on the question of Eddie's going home, Bill asked him if he would like to have some laundry done. Eddie said he would and then blurted out, "But I'll look goofy walking around with my shirt all wrinkled like those little kids do." It then became clear that Eddie's primary reason for leaving was that he was running out of clothes and would lose face in front of the younger boys if he appeared dressed as they did.

Bill secured an iron, and one of the female counselors offered to iron Eddie's shirts for him. From this point on, adults in the camp were "okay" in Eddie's terms and he stayed until the end of the camping session.

Younger children will often initiate or suggest a competitive dressing activity themselves. The counselor's role here should be somewhat low-keyed, making it easier for the winner or loser to be forgotten and for the completion of the task to be the most rewarding thing for the child. Sometimes, children will pair up in competition against the counselor. For example, two youngsters will delay while the counselor is waiting for them to signal him to begin counting, and all the time they are delaying, they are getting dressed. They would then suddenly appear fully dressed and in the hall when the counselor began at the count of one. Here, they had used the motivation of the game to complete the task, but were less dependent upon the counselor in carrying it through. Some children seem to need a counselor in the bedroom to help them control the external stimulation present at this time. The mere presence of the counselor might create a new problem and it is wise to put some activity between yourself and the child. For example, one counselor was successful in using simple games of skill during this period. She would encourage a child to throw a ball or a stuffed animal toward a large cardboard box; if the object landed in the box, the child would agree to put on one article of clothing. This would continue until the child was completely dressed and ready to go downstairs. That child would use the same game to undress in the evening time.

Some mornings, children are awake and running full tilt when the counselor arrives. There may have been some mild sex-play and the behavior had spread to the group. At such times, it is advisable to restore order surely and calmly by returning the boys to their rooms and re-establishing the routine while perhaps moving in a little more quickly to help the boys get dressed. We may have to insist on a child's getting dressed within a certain time limit. If necessary, one might change the location of the child to cut down on his stimulation and enable him to complete the task of dressing. For example, a child may be asked to dress in a bathroom or spare bedroom. On these occasions, it should be made clear to the child why he is placed in the room and what is expected of him while he is there. If the counselor observes carefully, and picks the right child to remove, the other children can often settle back reasonably soon to the tasks at hand.

Tim, the youngest child in the group, often would spend an excussive amount of time in getting dressed. At the same time, his masturbatory activities during this period would stimulate the other children to a frenzy of sexual excitement. (He often seemed bewildered, since this was not his express intent.) Attempts at interpreting to him the consequences of his behavior were of little avail. It was finally decided that he would dress in an adjoining room and then proceed downstairs as soon as he was finished dressing. This procedure cut down greatly on the contagion of his roommates.

During the dressing period, the counselor can do numerous things to show interest, to teach, or to help a youngster to feel at ease about the way he looks. A comb or a belt can be offered or overly long pants may be cuffed; the counselor might suggest that a certain shirt be buttoned or tucked in, or another one left out. It also is an excellent opportunity for the child-care worker to comment on the physical growth of the child in reference to the larger clothing sizes or shoe sizes that he is now using.

One final point on dressing routines. Many children who are in institutions become particularly attached to an article of clothing they brought from their own home or from a foster home. They may zealously guard this possession even when it has become tattered and threadbare, and counselors can help in this regard by making sure that the article of clothing is kept in reasonably good repair and is washed regularly. One should not be fooled into thinking that he is doing the child a favor by throwing such a ragged article away and presenting him with a new one.

Breakfast Routines

Food is a crucial medium of exchange in the therapeutic milieu, one that is especially important at this early part of the day. Children have now moved from their bedrooms to the larger living spaces downstairs. There may be a small cluster in front of the television set, some others may be preparing for school, others may be enlisting the aid of a counselor, having developed an elaborate set of rules governing the seating arrangements in front of the television set, the order in which boys may cook breakfast, and the like. Generally, when the children are watching cartoons (no *Three Stooges* allowed) and seem in no immediate hurry to eat, the counselor will often sit with them, enjoying a cup of coffee, and offer quiet suggestions as to what the children might like for breakfast. This rather subtle competition with *Popeye* takes effect after a while and the children place orders, while some of them begin to prepare their own breakfast.

If two counselors are on duty, one should probably be in the kitchen and dining area, the other assisting the late risers upstairs. One counselor has made particularly good use of the kitchen at such times. Some children may be engaged in a quiet conversation while breakfast is being prepared. Another child who has had difficulty in the group may be asked to sit quietly at the table until the counselor can be with him. Occasionally, a counselor may place construction paper and scissors on the table for a child who likes to do simple craft work while waiting for breakfast or for school. On particular mornings, he may have three or more children sitting in various positions around the kitchen, all the time carrying on a running conversation with them, perhaps even trying to resolve some problem. The counselor may be simultaneously working with the total group, and handling individual problems that arise while preparing breakfast.

As a general rule, children are expected to be indoors until after breakfast. It is very difficult for some children to get back into breakfast after they become engaged in an outside activity. Counselors have found that suggestions of pre-breakfast activities, eliciting suggestion of breakfast choices, and things of this nature will tend to keep children occupied until after they have eaten. There may be exceptions to this rule.

Toby almost always woke up fighting. He would begin his attack on his roommate; this would often spread to the counselors on duty and some of the other children. Mary, his counselor, suggested that perhaps he could use some time alone at this period and away from the group. This was virtually impossible to accomplish within the cottage. He was allowed to go outdoors within a limited space to swing or climb a tree before breakfast. Before he left, the counselor would get his breakfast order and this would act as somewhat of a lure to get him back into the cottage. Of course, the counselor had to deal with the objections of other boys who were not allowed outside privileges at this time. She explained that Toby had problems in being around others before breakfast, and it was important for him to be by himself. At the same time, she made an effort to engage the others in some interesting cooking and crafts activities in the house so that they would not feel they were missing out on anything.

One function of limiting the child's life space at this time of the day is that children may be kept close to adults, right up until school time. The counselor can become aware more quickly of moods and particular problems of a child and can handle these before school. Thus, the child has a better chance of succeeding in the morning session. Also, the children seem to need preparation before they move to the larger social area of the school. Children present a wide range of idiosyncrasies around breakfast time and the management techniques of the child-care worker must be individualized and flexible to fit the needs of a particular child within the larger framework of the larger routine. Some examples might demonstrate such flexibility.

Elias would often awake during the night because of a frightening nightmare. An early riser, he easily became a crabby, grumpy child and was often a scapegoat for the other children. Mary, his counselor, found it wise to approach him early and to engage him in the reality of the new day. His best mornings occurred when he got dressed quickly and became involved in cooking his own breakfast. Techniques such as humor could work well with Elias in getting him through the different stages of the morning routine.

Ricky, on the other hand, was loathe to become engaged with any adults or children in the morning. His counselor, Bill, would come on the shift and find him going full tilt, lashing out at adults and children. Bill found that the best "solution" to Ricky's morning problems were preventative steps that could be taken the night before: a comic book left on the bedside table for Ricky to read the next morning or a game left on his shelf that he could play with if he woke up early. Mornings when Ricky was already off and running, Bill often found that the thing that worked best was simply to give Ricky some space. Ricky was allowed to leave the cottage and go outside.

Mike is a child who derives a good deal of support from the early morning routine, often following it flawlessly until school time. However, if something goes amiss in the routine, Mike may regress fairly quickly into some very infantile behavior. This regression can be stopped rather easily, however, by a firm word from the counselor. Motivation to get through the morning routine for Mike centers largely around breakfast. Cooking one of his specialties, deluxe scrambled eggs, often brings him out of his regressive stage to a point at which he is ready to deal appropriately with other children. This child uses numerous props to get through the early part of the day, food being one, certain television programs being another.

The following are a few suggestions about breakfast itself. Some children say they are not hungry, or simply refuse to eat. In such cases, it often helps to suggest a fairly stock item that children can have any time: tea and toast, milk and toast, hot chocolate. Somehow this suggestion lessens the resistance of coming to breakfast as the children see it more as a snack than as a meal. Counselors have developed a cut-off point, after which boys may not participate in making their own breakfast. Beyond this point, the child may have cereal, fruit, or toast.

Breakfast provides a good opportunity to sit with the children and to discuss with them the general outline of the day itself. Not infrequently one finds the child who simply refuses to eat anything at this time of day. Generally speaking, no one will make a fuss about this. Given the amount of food that is available to all of the children during the course of the day and given the fact that sooner or later, the child is going to become hungry and want something to eat, it is not worth while to make a "big thing" about his not eating at this time.

Generally, breakfast can be looked upon as a test run for the later morning experiences of the child. It is, in fact, one of the first social situations of the day and counselors may use it as a test situation to help determine which children they should be watching closely during the course of the particular morning.

Fred would come downstairs and, when asked by his counselor what he wanted for breakfast, he would often reply "nothin' " in a very disgusted voice. Usually, this meant that some issue had remained unsolved from the night before, usually something that had to be settled before Fred could move on to school or any other program activity.

In short, breakfast can be an important relationship building time that will give the child-care worker some management leverage he is likely to draw upon later in the morning.

Moving Off To School

At this point in the routine counselors begin to make more explicit demands upon the children. Simply because of the time factor involved, reminders about finding coats and shoes and finishing breakfast will increase during this period. It is therefore crucial for the children to be aware continually of the amount of time until the school session begins. To announce suddenly that it is now time for school, with no forewarning, can be disasterous. Often children can be literally led to school in Pied Piper fashion by engaging them in interesting, short-term activities that end up at the school door. These activities inevitably will approximate the model of "Follow the Leader" with many variations.

Sometimes, a child will prefer to go to school early to show a teacher a crafts project or something he completed the night before. A more directed game or activity close to school time will help the child gear into the directions and demands that will be placed upon him in the classroom. If the child begins to suggest long-term projects before school, the counselor suggests that after school might be a better time, indicating the lack of time for successful completion of the project as well as the difficulty of getting to school on time. Children may also exhibit many of the somatic complaints that were witnessed at bedtime the night before. These are dealt with in a calm, reassuring, but not overly concerned fashion. At this time probably more than at any other time in the morning routine, the counselor is forced to make rather quick and decisive judgments as to whether a particular child should be allowed into the classroom. Some examples here might be helpful.

Dale had a rather poor morning and it was now time for school. He had had several scuffles with his peers and was in such a phase of heightened activity that his counselor felt it would not be wise to send him to school without first finding out what the trouble was. Dale balked at this, saying, "If I don't get to go to school now, I ain't gonna do no work for the morning."

Finally, when the other boys had left, Dale began to sob. He told the counselor that this was to be his day to work with a student teacher at school on his reading problem. Dale blurted out that the student teacher had suggested that they use a tape recorder and in that way they would be able to listen to Dale's voice in order to help him with his reading. The counselor asked him if he had ever done this before and he said, "No."

What quickly came to light, then, was that Dale was very frightened of entering into this project with the student teacher. He thought that his voice would sound "funny" on the tape, and he really didn't want to record it. However, this was an activity all the other boys regarded as quite positive and gratifying and he felt that it would seem stupid if he made a fuss about not wanting to work with the tape. Dale's counselor called school on the intercom, and together she and the student teacher discussed Dale's problem in his program for the morning. The student teacher made it clear that this was not something Dale had to do but, in fact, something he might want to do after listening to some other things on the tape. Dale went to school shortly thereafter.

Here was an example of a problem that almost needed to be worked through before the child could arrive at school. Many times we send a child to school with the knowledge that the routine of school, the presence of the teacher, and the presence of a task will be enough to bind up any problems he might be having at the moment.

Timmy had been buzzing around the group rather constantly before breakfast. It was a Monday morning and he had had a particularly rough weekend with two of his roommates. There appeared to be some legitimate question as to whether Tim could attend school that morning. His counselor, John, felt that we should try it, stating Tim's very positive relationship with the teacher and the fact that he had had some difficulties with two particular boys over the weekend. We decided to let him go, and all the way to school, Tim was making rather joking threats about what he was going to do, "Tear the place up, bust a window." As soon as he crossed the threshold of the school, however, he hung up his coat and became engaged in the activity of the morning session.

Here, the child saw the school as a welcome change from the demands of the cottage life and was actually eager to get there. A decision to keep him back from the school program would probably have triggered off a major blow-up.

Summary

We have seen, then, that wake-up time requires that the child shift from a primary awareness of an investment in himself and begin dealing with the outside world. To aid in this task, we have provided individualized help within the structure of the overall routine, which is directed at aiding the child to cope with the problems he encounters early in his day and to teach him some new ways of handling these problems. We depend upon rules, routines, and activities, plus our relationship with the child, to provide assistance to him in making this necessary shift.

Rules should be rather simple and direct and should, in effect, save the child from the necessity of dealing excessively with other children or with adults to gain his rights or prerogatives. For example, we have a rule about assigned seats in front of the television for early-morning viewing which has alleviated the problem of children feeling they have to negotiate who sits where. At times, this is something we might want to have the group do, but at this time of the morning, it is a problem we would rather do without.

Similarly, all of the routines are supportive in the sense that they provide a framework within which the child can progress from his earliest waking phase until the time he gets ready for school. For instance, clean clothing is laid out for each child at the same time of day; things like tooth brushes, tooth paste, and soap are always available for use. Some of the informal routines we have previously described, such as the informal chatting that goes on between counselor and child in the morning, are a very integral part of the day for many children. As the routines progress through the morning period, they allow a greater latitude to the child in terms of what he wants to do for himself. For instance, the breakfast routine includes the possibility of a child's selecting food and cooking his own breakfast in its entirety or allows him merely to place his order and have the counselor prepare his breakfast much as he desires. We have found that the existence of a time schedule for the tasks of the morning and the repetitiveness of the schedule along with clear expectation patterns of just what the events of the morning program will be have tended to be a very useful aid to our children in coping with the problems of early morning.

One of the other positive functions of a strong routine, is that it takes the onus of limit setting off a completely personalized basis. When a child is asked to stop an action, he is asked to do so because the behavior is not acceptable, not because of the counselor's own idiosyncrasy but rather because it is a part of the code of the institution.

Activities provide a third very important aid in helping to control the child in the life-space. These should be simple and not too demanding, activities that focus the child on the adult rather than on other children usually work best. This is not the time for mass activities. When used in conjunction with a particular part of the routine—for example, the dressing routine—a simple game such as timing of various parts of the process can be very helpful in getting the child to the stage where he is ready to leave the bedroom area and to eat breakfast. Finally, the counselor may use activities to move children from place to place in the milieu. For example, he may use a Follow-the-Leader game to aid children in going from the cottage to the school. While it is one of the shortest periods of time that we have to manage during the day, this early morning phase can be crucial to the child's progress for the rest of the day. In contrast to bedtime, where we are attempting to slowly ease the child out of the social realm, getting him to relax his defenses and get ready for sleep (Trieschman, Paradise, and Segal 1967), in the morning, we are bringing the child back into the world of his peers, back into contact with adults, and back into situations like school, where demands are going to be made upon him. It is important, therefore, that through the use of rules, routines, and activities, we provide support where it is needed but also allow the child the opportunity to cope with some of these problems on his own.

References

BETTELHEIM, BRUNO. 1950. From dreams to waking. In *Love is not enough*. Glencoe, Ill.: Free Press.

REDL, FRITZ. 1966. What do we do about the facts of life? In *When we deal with children*. Glencoe, Ill.: Free Press.

———, and DAVID WINEMAN. 1957. *The aggressive child*. Glencoe, Ill.: Free Press.

TRIESCHMAN, A. E., R. J. PARADISE, and R. L. SEGAL. 1967. Bedtime management in a children's home. This volume and *Mental Hygiene*, 51(2): 209–220.

V

MANAGING MEALTIME BEHAVIOR

Albert E. Trieschman
James K. Whittaker

Mealtime provides unique opportunities for close work between the children and the child-care staff of the residential treatment unit. Eating is often associated with close familial groupings sitting in comparative quiet around a table, discussing plans, sharing concerns, and enjoying each other's company. Even in "normal" families, however, there is much variation, particularly in regard to the role played by the children. The range of experiences and the attitudes associated with mealtime increases considerably where some members are disturbed. In such families mealtime may be the emotional low spot of the day as interaction between parents and children are heightened due to the forced proximity of the dining area. Rather than being looked forward to eagerly, mealtime may be anticipated with dread. Social histories record a multitude of scenes around the kitchen table where parents fight with each other and with the children. Favoritisms and rivalries are often dramatically acted out, and in the broken home missing parent's absence is dramatically brought into focus at each meal. While much consideration has been given to the patho-

This chapter was prepared with the help of Robert J. Paradise.

logical symptoms in relation to eating, surprisingly little has been written about the management of mealtime behavior in an institutional setting. In our discussion of the therapeutic utilization of mealtime in the treatment residence we shall focus particularly on the management issue.

The staff of an institution—particularly the child-care workers who are physically closest to the children—are usually aware of the meaning of food and mealtime to a child almost immediately upon the child's arrival. Their reports of the child's first meal often describe his refusal to come to the table. If he does come, they report such things as fighting with other children, refusal to eat, overeating, lack of "manners," requests for a great deal of food but consumption of very little, fear of asking for food to be passed, playing with food, or bizarre manipulations of food and utensils. Some of this behavior can be attributed, initially, to the fearfulness engendered by eating with a group of strangers; but most of this difficult behavior is possible any time that a group of emotionally disturbed children are gathered together in the treatment residence's dining room.

In this paper we will consider first the task facing the child at mealtime. For convenience we have divided the tasks into three parts: (1) the transition from activities to sitting down at the table; (2) food—its meaning and acceptance, handling and passing it, and using utensils; (3) ending the meal. Following the discussion of these tasks, we will describe some areas of therapeutic management available to the adults at the table. The tasks involved in mealtime and the management techniques we will describe are drawn largely from our experience at Walker Home with character-disordered latency-aged children. The third section will deal with management of mealtime behavior, and the final section will outline a number of suggestions found to be useful by our child-care staff during mealtimes.

Tasks of Mealtime

The common, everyday act of eating a meal is actually a complex act, particularly for the ego-defective child. Its difficulties are heightened or exaggerated in many ways in the residential treatment setting because of the presence of other disturbed children, to mention only the most obvious difference between the institution and home.

While mealtime might abound with therapeutic possibilities, getting the child to the table may represent a major achievement in and of itself. The first task, then, is that the child must stop the pleasurable activity he may be involved in as the bell rings. This is made more difficult because the stopping is necessitated by adult reasoning. It is not always that the child is hungry—it is rather that the staff has meals prepared at particular hours.

The activity a child is being asked to leave might be an exciting game of baseball or an interesting conversation with the maintenance man. In neither case will the child come to the table as soon as he hears the bell. The child-care worker is often greeted with, "So what? I'm not hungry" or "You go ahead, I'll be there in a couple of minutes." What we think of as an intrinsically rewarding activity becomes a full-scale management struggle. The child-care worker will be wise if he avoids making a deliberate "issue" out of coming to meals and rather uses the various transition time activities (see Chapter III, p. 107) and games (see Chapter IV, pp. 131–135) to move the children from one routine to another. While we generally strive for flexibility in our institutional program, we feel the regularity of mealtimes is helpful in that it represents a stable "landmark" around which the child can orient himself three times daily. Schedules, carefully planned with this in mind, become a part of the therapeutic milieu. This reassurance of regular feeding, often in sharp contrast to the child's prior experience, offers much in the way of emotional support. The interchangeability between *food* and *love* in our culture adds support to the positive aspects of feeding children in treatment.

The transition from school or activity to dinner is still a difficult one; between the time a child leaves a ball game and walks into the dining area, he may be involved in one or more scuffles and be subjected to the seduction and lure of a thousand different stimuli along his path. Games, as mentioned earlier, are particularly useful, especially those of the "Follow-the-Leader" variety. There are also certain structures and rituals we can use to help bridge this transition time. For example, play equipment is put away, coats are hung up in the same place, hands are washed, and children are toileted; all of these acts serve as "markers" which tell the child that the activity is over and the meal is about to begin. Because of their habitual nature, these acts may serve as external controls to the child who feels some anxiety about entering a crowded dining room. It is important that the child go into the dining hall feeling protected and capable of following directions from the counselor. The rambunctious, unresponsive child is kept from the dining hall until ready to enter, as his own poor controls will surely disintegrate in the close setting. Counselors should be right with the children at this time, directing and controlling the flow of behavioral traffic. Sitting down at the table is an act that is both physically and psychologically difficult for our children to manage. This difficulty is often magnified by having to wait for food to be served or passed and by the presence of other children who may represent a threat. The typical social mechanisms that serve to allay pre-meal anxieties are often denied to the disturbed child; thus, the immediate events of the day may have been too "painful" to utilize as table talk. This, in addition to the fact that "talking" is not usually a characteristic way for the impulsive, hyperaggressive child to handle anxiety. The major responsibility for helping the child ward off the stresses at this point in the meal falls to the child-care worker. He accomplishes this by seeing that food is served quickly, that the individual tastes of the children are taken into account, and that the children are reassured as to the adequacy of the food supply.

The second task faced by the child at mealtime involves accepting, handling, passing, and eating food. For some children the act of accepting food itself signals a great deal of anxiety. Issues of dependency on the adults are raised anew; the very philosophy of the milieu described in terms of "giving," "nurturing," and "accepting" are highlighted when the child must accept food from the adult. Essentially the child is asking, "You are giving me all of this—what are you going to demand in return?" To children who may have experienced the manipulation of food as punishment or as a bribe for parental affection, the fantasy of what will be demanded by the giving child-care worker may be somewhat frightening. Many newly arrived children either eat very little or refuse to eat at all on their first day in the residence. Some children choose to skirt this issue by refusing to eat at mealtimes but gorge themselves at snack time or when they are allowed to buy food outside of the residence. Both are examples of situations where children can feed themselves. This is acted out another way when a new child insists on bringing food to the table and feeding himself.

Food and utensils often represent a powerful stimuli to disturbed children; we are all too familiar with the child who impulsively siezes a knife or fork and makes mock threats toward another child. We are often less sensitive to the lure of other table utensils; thus, a pitcher of milk or a pepper shaker is overlooked, though we would be extremely cautious about leaving a bucket of paint or a can of talcum powder near the same child! Associations and double entendres to common mealtime words ("meat," "hot dog," "peas") may be enough to contage an entire group. This does not mean that these foods are never served, only that the staff is alert to the seductions that are likely to go along with them. New and strange foods are often greeted with epithets and disdain; the child-care worker should attempt to explain the new dish but not make the mistake of trying to "oversell" it.

The final task facing the child is that of ending the meal. For some children a rewarding table game may terminate in a regressive food orgy with the leftover table scraps. Some children just naturally take a long time to finish a meal, while others are often through before the counselor has taken his first bite. The skillful use of table games, conversation, and mealtime routines will help reduce the time gap between these two. A child may leave the dining hall when he has finished his meal and when he is excused by a counselor; however, he may not re-enter the dining hall and this often presents a problem.

Jerry would often bolt his meal and ask to be excused first from the table. A mad dash to the living room or outside and he would re-enter muttering, "There's nothing to do out there." He would often attempt to disrupt the other youngsters by pulling their chairs or poking at them. Staff, with the aid of Jerry's tablemates, talked about the social as well as the nutritional benefits of mealtimes: talking with staff and children about future activities or past successes, participating in games, and just plain relaxing. With Jerry, staff worked out a special arrangement where he could begin to clear dishes and utensils immediately upon finishing his meal and then return to the table for dessert and conversation. This allowed him a relatively high degree of physical movement while still keeping him hooked into the routine.

Counselors make an attempt to mark the end of the meal as clearly as they marked the beginning. Thus, the boys must ask to be excused from the table. After the noon meal, they have five or ten minutes of cleanup chores in their bedrooms and living areas. To further accentuate the end of the meal, no food is allowed out of the dining room. Children are reminded of the time remaining until the next major event of the day ("School begins in thirty minutes") and are assisted in finding activities that will last roughly that amount of time. No pressure is placed on children to participate in games or activities, since many prefer to spend the transition time quietly reading or writing a letter home. Having now delineated the tasks a child faces at mealtime, we will proceed to a discussion of therapeutic management of mealtime behavior.

Therapeutic Management

The child-care worker has some very definite goals related to mealtime. He would like the children to come to the table and eat as much food as they need for adequate nutrition. He would like to eat his own meal. He would like all of this accomplished with a minimum of upset, disruption, and mess. He may be interested in teaching table manners and introducing new foods to the child's diet, or he may wish to use this time when several children are together to plan or discuss the day's activities including any recent problems the group has encountered. In order to achieve these goals, behavior must be reasonably well controlled at the table.

The role of the child-care worker in controlling behavior—the management techniques he applies—may be discussed in five separate but overlapping areas: *structure, rules, techniques for handling upsets, teaching "manners,"* and *the use of activities.*

Structure

Contagion can be a major problem at the table. In anticipation of this, careful consideration should be given to seating arrangements. Assigning groupings by tables is determined by how easily that grouping will be contaged, how supportive tablemates might be toward each other in positive ways, how the boys relate as a group, and the staff's interest in promoting a particular grouping. It may be, for example, that a particular youngster is being encouraged to assume more leadership among his peers. The table arrangement can be manipulated to maximize this opportunity.

The staff also needs to decide where a boy sits at a table: who must be within reach of a child-care worker, who is less provocative when next to his friend or perhaps across from his friend. We have noticed that the seating arrangement also aids management in a less direct way. The boys are well aware of why they sit in a particular seat and when a boy leaves the residence (a sign of health), the boy who moves into his seat achieves some of the departed boy's status and the expectations that go along with getting better. We see this happen even when most of the seats are rearranged to accommodate a new boy or a new situation.

Rules

Rules related to eating are generally not written down or codified. Rather, they are presented in the form of child-care worker "edicts"; that is, they represent the common table etiquette of a family. They are designed to reduce stimuli to which the boy is exposed during the meal. To begin with, unless boys are physically ill, they must come to the dining area even if they do not wish to eat. We explain this by pointing out that the staff must know where a boy is, to help or protect him, and that since the staff is eating, they cannot fulfill their part of the job if the child is not with them at the table. If a child is too upset to come to the dining area (due to anger or fear), a child-care worker stays with him until he is ready to come to the table. In these situations, the child often eats after the other boys have finished. In no case is a child deprived of a meal because he is upset.

Other "rules" have to do with shouting between tables, getting up from the table, and handling food. For some boys the child-care worker must do the serving and pouring. As each child becomes healthier, he will be able to handle a platter of food without taking everything or spilling or throwing the contents. Until that time, the child-care worker maintains control over the serving functions. Boys bring food to the tables, serving on a rotating basis. This is voluntary and no issue is made by the child-care worker if a boy does not want to serve. Group pressure may be used by the other boys in some instances. It is one way to "feed yourself" and most of the time boys are quite eager to do it.

The atmosphere at mealtimes is not one of strict discipline, yet the general tone is controlled and interest centers around the child-care worker.

Techniques for Handling Upsets

As we have already stated, our prime interest is in preventing upsets before they occur. In many instances, the retracing of a mealtime upset shows that it could have been prevented or that it should have taken place away from the table. In these cases we can see that cues during the transition period before the meal were not accurately read, or "loose ends" of problems which should have been dealt with away from the table were not settled. At Walker Home the surface management techniques described by Redl are very much in use. A somewhat greater emphasis may be placed, particularly at mealtime, on the use of the group. For example:

> Ben was having a hard time cutting his food and began to get wild. The child-care worker offered to help cut his meat but this made Ben even angrier. He shouted, "I'm not a damned baby! I'll do it myself; Keep away." The child-care worker turned to Jerry and suggested that he tell Ben how it was when he first came to the home. Jerry, and then Dan, began to talk about how they learned to do things and pointed out that counselors could teach and help boys. After the counselor had helped Ben cut his meat, the conversation stayed on the subject of how the boys had changed since coming to the home.
>
> On another occasion, Ted kept trying to get John excited by making motions of a sexual nature with his food and saying suggestive things to him. Neither boy responded to staff's suggestion to "cool it." Both were getting high. Staff pointed out what was happening and then posed the problem to the group at the table. "What's going to happen if you guys keep this up? Everyone will get excited and out of control; some guys will have to leave the table; no one will be having much fun after lunch. What are you going to do about it?" Alan told Ted to stop and the other boys joined in pointing out that they were going to work on the fort as soon as they were through eating and that Ted was "just trying to start trouble."

When it is necessary to remove a boy from the table, we have found that it is not always easy to decide which boy to "bounce." Since most of the acting-out at mealtime is of a contagious nature, there is often a choice between removing the instigator and the boy doing the acting-out. This is an important question because in the eyes of the group, the latter is seen as the "victim" and the former, who is often sitting innocently eating his meal, is known to the group as the true culprit. If the wrong boy is removed, it can be the signal for the entire group to act out.

Teaching

The primary purpose of teaching at the table is not the development of "prep school manners" but rather skills which will be ego-supportive. Thus, learning to ask someone to pass food instead of shouting for it, reaching across the table for it, or demanding it is not only the right way to do things, it is also the way that will produce the least stress and the least resistance in others. Another example is learning to use utensils, which may be more difficult than using fingers but which is less upsetting and stimulating. The sense of mastery, associated with the learning of ego skills, is related to the child's behavior and growth.

Our approach to teaching is flexible and is applied with little pressure. Before coming to the table, the boys wash their hands, although they often need and receive help in learning how to do this. The results, as with most latency-aged boys, often leave something to be desired. Rather than send a boy away from the table to wash again, the child-care worker must decide whether the boy's behavior controls will support his leaving the table and coming back. Often the decision is to ignore the soiled hands.

Much of the teaching is done by example; the child-care worker may over-emphasize the way in which he asks for something from the other end of the table, pointedly saying "please" and "thank you." Other things are taught as ritualistic games. For example:

> Mr. R. (a staff member who rarely ate with the boys) sat down at the table and began to eat. John had shouted, "Napkins!" Mr. R., not knowing what it was about, ignored it. I waited to see the boy's reaction. John said, very maturely, "Mr. R., don't you know you're supposed to put your napkin on your lap before you eat—you missed the signal." Everyone laughed.

Learning to eat with other people is something to do while at the table. Mastering skills becomes a way of reducing other stimuli, which also serves to meet needs by alleviating hunger more rapidly and efficiently and to ward off the attacks and provocations of others.

Activities

Another kind of learning that acts to reduce upsets is the use of activities at the dinner table. Again, the controls center on the child-care worker. The gap between the courses of the meal is filled with games to avoid the problems of delayed gratification and prolonged sitting. Word games are most frequently used by the child-care worker for two reasons: first, they require least movement and thus reduce motor activity which can be stimulating and exciting; second, they provide the opportunity to teach information and learning skills. To reduce frustration, games and activities are kept simple and competition is either absent or de-emphasized. For many months a popular game was one in which boys had to name animals whose initials would be given by another boy or a child-care worker. This game developed many variations and through it, the boys learned the differences between mammals, reptiles, etc., as well as an enormous number of animal names. Number games were used in the same way, and some have been created by our school staff specifically for this purpose as an adjunct to what the boys are studying in school.

Storytelling is another popular activity and is especially useful when it is important to center attention on the child-care worker and reduce activity among the children to a minimum. Stories of earlier exploits and delinquent activities are used by the child-care worker to point out the reasons leading to the boys' coming to the home for help and may be used to explain and give insight into an event which took place earlier in the day. In some ways mealtime, more than any other situation during the day, gives the child-care worker a "captive audience" with the emphasis on the audience. Some of the discomfort of discussion, learning, and self-examination is balanced by the oral gratification the child receives. Often what happens at the table can only be compared to what one would expect to take place in group therapy. When this occurs, the optimum therapeutic use is being made of mealtime.

Suggestions

This section deals with a number of suggestions found to have been useful by child-care workers in dealing with mealtime behavior.

1. The child-care worker can "teach" the routine of a meal largely by modeling the correct behavior himself. This is easier said than done. Child-care workers are rushed, tired, and often at an emotional low point around mealtimes. An overattention to our own nutritional needs may elicit anxious responses from the youngsters. Thus, we should make an attempt to model commonly accepted table etiquette and be sure not to begin our own meals until the children have been served.

2. The counselor should pass out the food to each individual child to ensure that each one gets started on his meal. It is often too much to bear for the child who has had difficulty with the group all morning to have the other children "touching" his food. There is also a good deal of seductive value in a heaping plate of food in the hands of an impulse-disordered youngster, especially when the food belongs to someone else!

3. The dinner table should be cleared of all seductive gadgetry before the meal begins. Such items as drinking-straw wrappers, carving knives, large pot covers, breakable glassware, sharp objects, and unnecessary spices should be removed; they add nothing to the decor of the table and often provide a situational lure for the diners.

4. When children are entering the dining area, it is wise to have a counselor near each table so that the child is not wholly exposed to the contents of the entire meal.

> Ray plucked a piece of ham from the serving plate before the meal today and occasioned a collective burst of anger from the rest of the group. Joey cried, "I'm not going to eat after that 'pig' put his hands all over it!"

5. The alternative selections to the main dish should be determined before the meal; thus, something like "peanut butter and jelly" is always available for the child who does not care for the main meal. It has been our experience that not forcing a child to eat prevents an unnecessary management issue. If

a child is angry or in a sulk and refuses to come to the table, he may stay in a designated spot in the lounge until the meal is completed. His food will be saved a reasonable length of time and then the "universal alternative" (peanut butter and jelly) will be made available to him if he wishes.

6. Second helpings are generally something that should be determined in advance; there is no worse fate than being confronted by six children and eight pieces of chocolate cake. We must often repeat the policy of the institution for the new child, "We seldom have seconds on the main course, but always on milk, bread, etc."

7. Seating plans should be assigned and not left to the individual choices of the children. This rather undemocratic suggestion is based on our observation that children have enough to deal with mealtimes without the added burden of deciding where to sit. This plan also allows us to manipulate a rather important variable, the child's position vis-à-vis the group and the child-care worker. Thus, the newer younger children who will require the most assistance sit within easy reach of the counselor. An added benefit is that a child's place at the table becomes "his territory" and serves to mark the routine for him in a tangible way.

8. As a general rule, it is best to have the child-care worker and not the kitchen staff monitor the amounts of food given to each child. Each cook is bound to have her "favorites" and woe be the day when Johnny ends up with the extra scoop of ice cream or extra piece of pie. Counselors should eat the same meals as the children, albeit in slightly larger proportions.

9. Counselors should always be aware of their own table etiquette; smoking, for example, may be especially bothersome to some younger children and wholly intolerable to older adolescents who are denied the privilege. Similarly, this is *not* the time to read personal mail or become engaged in clinical conversation "over the heads of the children."

10. Finally, we have found it almost universally true that most latency-aged children require some sort of short, total body activity after meals. This might be a brief game of catch or tag, or a short ride on a bicycle. This is often a difficult

suggestion to follow (and becomes increasingly so the older you get!), but it becomes extremely important to provide some sort of carryover between the meal and the activity and/or routine that is to follow.

References

LONG, NICHOLAS J., and RUTH G. NEWMAN. 1965. Managing surface behavior of children in school. In Nicholas J. Long, William C. Morse, and Ruth G. Newman (Eds.), *Conflict in the classroom*. Belmont, Calif.: Wadsworth.

VI
MANAGING BEDTIME BEHAVIOR

Albert E. Trieschman

Private schools, summer camps, group foster homes, and residential treatment centers all face the problem of helping groups of children go to bed and to sleep. We have focused on helping child-care workers to plan their management actions with children. They are the adults who have maximum contact with the children and who largely determine the therapeutic effectiveness of the milieu.

We have chosen bedtime for discussion because it is common to all residential group settings and because it so often presents problems. The difficulties of getting children to bed and to sleep have become a cultural cliché. The cartoon of the harried, tense adult faced with a child who demands yet another glass of water is all too familiar. Recourse to antitherapeutic actions by the managing adult (often actions that increase fear in an already frightened child) are frequent. Trying to do "psychotherapy"—i.e., talking to a child about the difficulty—is at best a partial solution. Staff coverage is inadequate for this one-to-one process, and prolonged conversations at bedtime tend to obviate the necessity for going to

This chapter is adapted from an earlier journal version. Trieschman, A. E., R. J. Paradise, and R. L. Segal. 1967. Bedtime management in a children's home. *Mental Hugiene,* 51(2): 209–220.

sleep. Institutional routines at bedtime often seem designed more for institutional efficiency than for teaching adaptive behavior to an individual child or to a group of children. In short, it seems to us that bedtime is a child-management situation particularly suited to a demonstration of the usefulness of new thoughts on the therapeutic use of a milieu.

The staff of Walker Home has developed a network of ideas about the management of children that serves as a background to our discussion of bedtime. Teaching and learning are the central ideas in our conceptual framework for the therapeutic management of behavior. Alternative behavior is what we are teaching: our patients are learning alternatives to their sick behavior. Altering behavior includes (1) the interruption of disturbed or disturbing deviant behavior, and (2) the substitution of more adaptive, age-appropriate behavior based on ego skills. The substituted behavior may be really new to a particular child or it may be already familiar behavior that the child has never used in a particular situation.

We have found it helpful to think of our efforts to alter behavior in terms of three processes: reward and punishment learning, imitation-identification learning, and insight learning. To some extent we can choose to teach by these processes. We design rewards for some behavior and punishments (lack of rewards, restriction of privileges) for other behavior; we offer our behavior as a model for the children and ourselves as people with whom they can identify.

However, as therapeutically oriented adults, we prefer insight as a means of teaching. It avoids the damage to relationships likely to occur with reward and punishment and promotes ego strength, rather than feeding primitive, punitive superego behavior modulation, as reward and punishment are apt to do. Explanations and insights tend more to produce generalized knowledge about self, knowledge that will be more transferable to other situations than either identification-imitation or reward and punishment learning.

But we do need to manage situations long before we are in a position to teach alternative behavior through insights and explanations. This is all the more apparent when the children in a particular group are selected for their defective ego structures. The pre-delinquent or character-disordered child is usually unable to reflect on his difficulties. The impulsive acting-out of this child is often dissociated or disowned. At other times, the attention called to the behavior may cause a relentless character assassination, directed at the adult or the child himself. This extreme superego reaction is pathological, but it is different only in degree from the way many latency-age children react to explanations of their behavior with, "I'll be good next time." In short, all children in this age group learn about themselves and alter their behavior on the basis of all three of the learning processes.

We need to be aware that one or a combination of these processes of learning is going on as we manage the children. The important issue here is our awareness of the processes and our attempts to balance their use. The children also learn from one another, and this learning goes on by these same processes. Awareness of the different learning processes helps us to control their use among the children (e.g., bullying); we try to minimize or maximize the possibility of a particular child's being a model for another child (e.g., by room arrangements, shower schedules); we urge children to explain their feelings and behavior to other children in ways that promote insight.

Awareness of the learning process is only the beginning of therapeutic management. The choice of the form of the "lesson" is very important, and one that is more in our control. By form we mean how our attempt to teach alternative behavior is packaged. We can package our lessons in a therapy session, in a rule, in a conversation at the dinner table, in the choice of a game, or in the planning of a series of activities. Thinking of the milieu as a learning situation, with processes and forms, helps us integrate therapy, program planning, and handling of children into a cohesive effort.

We first present a set of descriptive categories for the deviations in bedtime behavior, which range from normal naughtiness to distinctly pathological behavior. We also offer an analysis of group and individual ego functioning at bedtime. The adaptive behavior we should like to teach is based on our understanding of the ego's tasks at bedtime and on our knowledge of the sources of ego strength. Finally, we describe the Walker Home bedtime routine, which is a sample of our attempts to use a milieu therapeutically.

Deviations in Behavior at Bedtime

The range of "naughty," disturbed, or disturbing behavior of children at bedtime is magnificent in its breadth and variety. Aches and pains, loose teeth just discovered, drinks of water, temporary hallucinations, bizarre sexual identifications, and tears of anger and sadness all appear.

Our goal is to devise descriptive categories for bedtime behavior that will aid adults in managing children. At the outset we need accurate "surface" or "clinical" pictures of the behavior. What does it look like, sound like, and feel like? Is that "aggressive" child angry with an adult, a larger child, a smaller child, himself, or the world? Does he use his words, his hands, his feet, his possessions (throwing toys), or stony silence to express his fury?

We must avoid our tendency to describe behavior in terms of its guessed-at meanings—not because meanings are unimportant, but because having only meanings (i.e., losing the behavioral description) clouds management. It is certainly more difficult to invent a management technique for a child's "anger" than it is to invent a technique for managing his kicking other boys when showers are announced. There is a lesson in this mundane point: We are never in a position to "cure a child's anger"; at best we can help him to understand his anger (the meaning of his behavior) and to manage and direct its expression (teach him age-appropriate alternative behavior).

The creation of a planned series of steps at bedtime is a prerequisite to the identification of deviant behavior. The explicitness of the steps in the routine highlights the individual difficulties in coping with what is required. If what is required by the routine is a reasonably flexible version of ego processes, then some failures of ego (some deviant behavior) become more salient to the managers of the routine and to the children as well.

The first descriptive category for deviant behavior at bedtime, then, is its *location in the bedtime routine*. This requires distinguishing between behavior that operates against getting into bed and behavior that operates primarily against getting to sleep. The child whose bedtime difficulties really begin when he has to stop a pleasurable evening activity presents a different management problem from the child who needs an endless succession of drinks and trips to the bathroom after he is bed. Playing radios, talking, and putting lights back on are all mild examples of behavior directed against sleep. The avoidance of taking off clothes or promoting a fight are, by contrast, examples of behavior directed against getting into bed. Refinements of this category depend, in part, on the detail of the bedtime routine. The moments of undressing, or bathing, or putting the lights out are obvious demarcations in bedtime routines. The knowledge of when and where a child's deviant behavior appears in a series of activities is an important first step in planning therapeutic management.

The second descriptive category involves identifying the *locus among people* of the deviant bedtime behavior. Does it involve a group, adults, only one child, or some combination of these? The highly contagious nature of anxious, silly behavior at bedtime makes this category imperative. At whom is the behavior directed? Is the child seeking vicarious impulse discharge through exciting a number of children? Would he like to get an adult to himself, or does he want to put something or someone between himself and a helping adult?

Sometimes, of course, deviant behavior may not involve any "others." A child may stare quietly out of a darkened window and slowly but painfully become the victim of his own projected anger in the shape of a scary monster. The counselor needs to vary his actions in order to take into account whether the child scares others with his monster, denies the monster and provokes a fight, or manages his anxiety by trying to frighten an adult.

One aspect of the locus category that is easy to overlook is origin. We need to find out where the behavior originates.

The child who "fusses" the most is not necessarily the originator of the behavior. His own ego may have been penetrated or caused to malfunction by another child's "quieter" behavior (e.g., one child's whispering some "dirty" words to another who gets "excited" by this). Both children, in this case, need therapeutic management, i.e., need to learn some alternative behavior, with the counselor's help.

A third important aspect of bedtime deviations is accurate description of the *mode of expression*. At a minimum this requires distinguishing between verbal and physical deviations. Beyond this we should like to have distinctions as to the parts of the body (feet, hands, genitalia) or the things (e.g., teddy bears or cups) that may be involved. A general assessment of the tempo of the behavior (slow, preoccupied, and withdrawn versus vigorous, driven, or manic behavior, for example) also aids counselors to make adjustments in their management.

These three descriptive categories—location in the routine, locus among people, and mode of expression—constitute prerequisites to planning management.

Placing bedtime behavior deviations in the remaining two descriptive categories, developmental or psychosexual level of behavior and predominant mechanism of defense, is often difficult to do on the basis of a single aspect of behavior. But, if we are to manage therapeutically, we usually need to have a hypothesis about the developmental level involved in the behavior and about what ego process or ego fragments (defense mechanisms) a child is using. We need this information to help the child understand the issue with which he is grappling (Can he trust an adult? Will he be nurtured? Will he have control of his bodily processes?).[1] And we need this information to design alternative behavior that employs, if possible, the ego fragments the child still has available.

Of course, the accumulation of information in these categories provides the managing adults with an ongoing, fine-

[1] One could express these issues in the shorthand of psychosexual stages—oral, anal, phallic, etc.—but we have found it more useful to the managing adults to employ a variety of questions that express the tasks of emotional development at these stages.

grained, diagnostic picture of the child. Counselors need to learn something of these categories, and they become more comfortable working with disturbed behavior as they learn them. With this knowledge they also gain in capacity to make inefficient behavior visible and more understandable to the child and to help him learn alternatives.

Let us consider some examples of the usefulness of the *developmental level category* as it applies to bedtime deviations. The primitive and impulsive behavior that children display at bedtime includes the oral, anal, phallic, and oedipal—and their variants. Autoerotic activities (rocking and infantile masturbation), exposure of genitalia, toilet play, spitting, hostile flatulence, sex play, smearing activities—all seem to have a greater prominence among our children at bedtime.

Accurate assessment of the developmental problems involved has sometimes revealed that a child suffers a "deeper regression" and a more profound sense of loss at bedtime than at any other time in his daily activities. On occasion we have found that the developmental problems involved are the same ones that interfere with daytime activities. Noting these differences and similarities can be crucial to the counselor's therapeutic handling of the situation. Special preparation in the form of slight alterations in routine, focused conversations with a child, or the invention of special anxiety-binding activities (e.g., a game with a roommate) is often helpful to the child for whom bedtime arouses especially primitive developmental issues. Counselors find themselves unable to use their own ego and ego-teaching skills to bind these children's impulse anxiety at bedtime unless they alter their usual daytime handling. On the other hand, the child who faces very similar daytime and bedtime psychosexual problems can be handled in much the same way at bedtime as he has been handled during the day. It might be added that signs of progress (e.g., going on to a more advanced stage of psychosexual development) often appear in bedtime conversations and behavior. For example, the child often reveals his growing trust in his acceptance of a bedtime snack and his request to be tucked in.

Bedtime deviations in terms of their *predominant mechanism of defense* are closely linked to psychosexual development. Often the first sign of special bedtime difficulties is a rather rapid deterioration in the level of a child's ego defenses. He may go from a discussion of a daytime aggravation over an unfinished project to the invention of burglars, witches, or bogey-men who menace his safety. The counselors' recognition of the child's "projection" as a change in defense is a signal to teach some alternative behavior. Can this child bind his anger with some more direct expression, or do we need to participate in the projection and help him invent "a make-believe burglar gun" or "a witch trap"?

Our recognition of the change in defensive posture and our description of the ego fragment or partial defense the child is employing help us design alternative behavior. Perhaps we can model the alternative after the defense he is already using (by inventing a foil to the projected creature, as in the example above); perhaps the counselor can help the child imitate another child's defense (a rommate's chronic complaining might do). Over a longer period of time the counselor may be able to establish with the child an insight into the choices he has of means of binding his impulse-anxiety. Arranging a daytime conversation about broken toys may lead the child to sense his own feeling of breaking apart at night and help him to participate with the counselor in daytime resolutions of the problem so that it will not carry over to bedtime. The child may even begin to use at bedtime reminders of the projects he might work on the next day as a constructive extension of his ego's capacity to bind anxiety.

Other defenses (or ego scraps) that we have often seen at bedtime include identification with the aggressor (using a blanket to dress as a ghost), denial (hiding, arguing about bedtime hour), and magical thinking (requesting sleeping pills, rituals of possession placement). Clearly there are many others, and many varieties.

Although bedtime behavior deviations can be categorized in ways that are useful, the child-care counselor cannot categorize each episode of "naughtiness" he encounters. Initially, he may be able to use only the more superficial descriptive categories, but careful use of this knowledge alone helps guide therapeutic management. Knowledge based on a child's application diagnosis or on past experience with him leads to expectations that reduce the complexity of categorizing behavior. The greatest reduction in complexity, however, comes with increasing familiarity with the individual child in the Walker Home.

No child's behavior encompasses the entire range of possibility. As we begin to know the individual child, we begin to be able to help him at the time and in the ways that are best for him. We do this by observing his deviations in terms of the categories we have described. We have found that some form of management-focused understanding of behavior is a vital part of using a milieu therapeutically, and these categories help us to view our management problems in the context of the living situation.

Ego Tasks and Ego Teaching at Bedtime

Bedtime is a transition time, a time between the last activity of the day and sleep. The ego tasks of bedtime begin with the ending of the last activity, and, as in all endings, there is the danger of a temporary weakening of controls. This is especially true near the end of the day, when both children and staff tend to be fatigued. Weakening (with the possible loss of impulse control) must not be confused with relaxing; with the latter, the child will have sufficient trust in the child-care worker to relax his watchfulness and, eventually, sleep.

For the child, the bedtime transition becomes a time when considerable ego strength is needed. Pleasant activities must end, and what is for many children the very unpleasant and frightening process of going to bed must begin. Not only must the children surrender activities, they must also withdraw from the adult-shared world, suspending fun and delaying gratifications until the next day. It is a situation that presents the disturbed child with many frustrations and opportunities for aggression. Clothing must be changed, showers taken, teeth brushed. For many disturbed children these are difficult tasks. Concern with privacy, exposure of body parts, and conformity to adult expectations make difficult what is often a pleasant situation and frequently turn it into a period of high resistance. The degree of disturbance can magnify the bedtime procedures, making them almost unmanageable for both child and staff. The possibility of an aggressive episode in which problems will be acted out increases.

The child on his way to bed is subjected to many potential stimuli that may make sleep difficult. Basically, the child's ego needs to withdraw its investment in external stimuli (events, activities) at the same time that it increases its tolerance for internal stimuli (bodily sensations, thoughts, fantasies). This is a complex task that all children have to learn in the course of growing up. We hope that they can learn this kind of "shifting" without encumbering the balance of psychic life. The habitually withdrawn child often falls asleep easily, but he is so predominantly geared to mastering internal stimuli that sleeping does not require a major shift for him. On the other hand, the hyperactive, aggressive child is often in flight from his difficulties with internal stimuli and has major problems in shifting inward in order to sleep.[2]

We gear our management help to the sources of stimulation and the shifting that getting to sleep requires. It may help to visualize a continuum of multiple stimuli that often combine. At one end are stimuli arising from sources external to the child; at the other, stimuli that come from within the child himself. In some situations the concept of the continuum is not sufficiently descriptive because the stimuli affecting the child appear to jump or "switch over" abruptly from external to internal, or the reverse. Projection is an example of such shifting. On the other hand, external forces, often quite real, can mount and a "resonance phenomenon" be set up as responsive notes within the child are struck. Accurate observation and evaluation are needed to determine what has taken place.

The child-care worker may have to address himself to the

[2] Our patients at Walker Home are predominantly hyperactive, aggressive children and need a great deal of help with "shifting inward" or slowing down in order to rest. Our experience suggests that they do better with the opposite shift (waking up) than do our withdrawn patients. But both groups need to learn new ego skills in order to shift ego energies without damaging psychic balance.

external stimuli, the internal, or both. His assessment must be accurate to be effective. Thus, in a situation in which a child approaches hysteria because his night light suddenly burns out, a judgment must be made as to whether the upset can be alleviated by regarding this as an external problem and simply replacing the bulb, or whether the anxieties and fantasies of the child that are screaming (sometimes literally) to be heard must be dealt with before the controls can be re-established. Bedtime anxiety relating to bed-wetting, control of erotic impulses, fantasies of death and destruction in sleep, and fear of the darkness are frequently encountered examples of internal stimuli.

The child-care worker is continually faced with the need to make assessments of the source of stimulation so that he can teach the child to cope with the threat and eventually relax sufficiently so that he can get to bed and to sleep. The matching of the teaching with the source of the stimuli and the particular pathological condition is essential and demands the utmost skill on the part of the managing adults. The task is complex: one must work to decrease external stimuli and, at the same time, increase the ego's tolerance of internal stimulation.

We see four factors that may aid in solutions: the relationship of the child-care worker to the child, the routine or sequence of events at bedtime, the child himself, and the group of children as an entity. All four contribute to various kinds of learning (rewards, insights, and imitations) through various means (conversations, rules, etc.).

The *child-care worker's relationship with the children* is the first and foremost source of bedtime ego teaching. Ministering to physical needs can be helpful. The child-care worker's assurance and concern are vitally important tools, and may be expressed verbally and through action. Quiet talk, making plans for the coming day (especially with a child who is not too sure that he will not die before he wakes), getting an extra blanket, handing out a bedtime snack, tucking the child in—all teach the child ways to deal directly with sources of stimuli and anxiety. In some instances the child-care worker may use his skills of interpretation and clarification to the same end. Essentially, he must offer warmth and assurance to the child.

However, there are situations in which the use of the counselor's particular skill and relationship with a child are strongly contraindicated. One such circumstance is when a child's fear of attack—perhaps sexual attack—is heightened by the darkness. The fact that he is lying down, that he is relaxing controls while physically close to a parent-like adult may argue against working with the child through the personal relationship. At such times the child-care worker may be in a better position to manage the child if he deals with him in a more "impersonal" way. He may choose to teach in terms of a Walker Home rule or to re-describe a piece of the bedtime routine, giving the reasons for it and the necessity for following it.

We move now to a consideration of the *routine* as a source of teaching solutions to bedtime problems. The overall structure of the pre-bedtime and bedtime procedures is, in effect, a planned piece of ego teaching. In the most simplified sense, it serves to regularize and structure the events of bedtime, to make the sequence predictable to both child and adult, thereby blunting the stimuli to which the child is exposed. The routine serves to reduce anxiety in the sense that bedtime becomes a structured event, although the structure is not a regimented one. Thus the children know that, no matter what occurs, evening activity will end by a specified time, showers may be taken during a definite period, snacks will be brought around after they are in bed, lights will go out, and a story will be read. The routine becomes a series of certain occurrences at a time when uncertainties abound.

The routine is also designed specifically to reduce stimuli. For example, the order of taking showers is arranged to reduce the possibility of contagion and even overstimulation and to make the right child-care worker available to the most needy boys at the right time. Although the routine minimizes external stimuli to some degree, it is also geared to teaching the children to manage internal stimuli. Thus the child-care worker is always there, passing out snacks (meeting oral needs), talking quietly to the boys (reassuring and planning ahead), and taking care of minor physical complaints or finding an extra blanket. The reading of a bedtime story serves an important function by partially supplanting internal fantasy and thought processes with the plot and details of the story. The snack in bed and the story-reading seem to combine to maximize the chances that the child's sense of his body and his awareness of thoughts will be pleasant.

The *child himself* may provide additional solutions to bedtime problems. This frequently happens, but may go undetected since there may be no verbal expression of the event. The boy who gets out of bed after the child-care worker has finished the evening's story and goes to get himself a glass of water may be quietly (and in an acceptable way) reassuring himself of the presence of protecting adults in the room nearby. The bringing to bed of a favorite stuffed doll or toy gun also exemplifies the child's seeking his own solutions, as do night lights, checking to make sure doors are locked, or reciting prayers.

At times, particularly with disturbed children, the attempted solution may be unacceptable to the adult or to other children. Counterphobic behavior, such as a provocative child's fearing attack from the adult and attempting to alleviate his anxiety by precipitating an attack, is not unusual. A similar example is the child who is afraid of his roommate and acts out in such a way as to get either himself or the roommate removed from the room. Withdrawal quickly into sleep is yet another solution some children attempt in coping with the problems of bedtime.

The fourth factor in which solutions to the stresses of bedtime may be found is the *group* itself. The tone or atmosphere of the group, often hours before bedtime, provides a rather accurate barometer of things to come. Excitement, overstimulation, aggression, and anxiety all feed from the group as a whole to its individual members. Child-care workers caught up in the frustration of the group find it difficult to change the tone. On the other hand, they "breeze" through an easy bedtime when spirits are good, but not too high, and things are running smoothly.

The routine may do much to counteract the tone of the group. At other times, the tone of the group may serve a similar function for the upset individual boy. Just as an upset group will quiet down for an interesting story, the anxious child may stop acting out when he finds the group unresponsive. At times he may even obtain reassurances from the group itself. We note this more frequently among the boys who have been longest in our care. They are able at times to offer assurance and even clarification to each other in much the same way the child-care worker does. At the same time, the group's ability to manage the routine serves to give assurance to the individual.

In summary, we find it helpful to think of bedtime in terms of ego tasks, sources of the ego's stimulation (internal, external), and the resources (relationships, routine, the child himself, the group) that we can utilize to teach age-appropriate alternative behavior to disturbed children.

An Example of Bedtime Management

The Walker Home bedtime routine is offered as a "case illustration." It is the product of our staff's awareness of behavior deviations and their use of ego teaching. Just as an individual therapy session is not detailed in a paper on the technique of therapy, so our bedtime procedures are not an automatically given product of our ideas about management. The counselor's work requires intelligent and flexible use of the management ideas. The possibility or advisability of an exact duplication of our bedtime procedures is hardly the point: our purpose is to illustrate the helpfulness of management-focused ideas in using a milieu therapeutically.

Stopping the evening activity

At 8:00 P.M. the child-care worker stops the evening activity. The method he uses is important. By helping children to accept the idea that the evening program is over, the child-care worker can bring activities to a gentle halt. As early as 7:30

the child-care worker has begun to anticipate with the children the nearing end of evening activity. This is accomplished by repeatedly noting the time, discouraging the start of a long game or new activity, using the last ten minutes of play time for cleaning up, or involving the children in discussion before the television goes off. After an especially stimulating activity a snack can be inserted at 7:45 to aid the children's slowing-down process. These management actions structure the processes of change and adaptation, which are necessary functions of the ego in making a transition. They also provide several points at which the slowing-down process might be taught.

The child-care worker definitely stops the activity by deed, e.g., turning off the television set. Such an action performs an ego task for the child and signals the start of a different activity. The child-care worker should make the stopping and starting explicit by such a statement as, "It is now time for showers." A routine will develop when these procedures are consistently repeated every night.

Nevertheless, it is still likely that the children will resist going to bed. The child-care worker can deal with this resistance in several ways: by talking of the good things of the day past and the day to come, by looking forward to the pleasant aspects of the routine to come (snacks, showers, and stories), by involving children in the next phase of the routine (helping to get snacks ready), by separating the routine into bits that the children's weakened egos can manage, or by simply identifying their resistance as anger, disappointment, and so forth (helping the children verbalize as an alternative to acting-out).

The ego task to be managed at this juncture is stopping one activity and beginning another. The child-care worker manages the more difficult aspects of this process for the child. Deviations may be anticipated because the activity change occurs at the beginning of the routine. Deviations here are dealt with by offering behavior for the child to imitate (adult actions), involving the child and rewarding him by the sharing of an adult task (preparing snacks), and so on.

We can observe the upsets that occur at this juncture more carefully by considering them in the light of the categories of deviation previously described. Denial, counterphobia, and infantilization may occur in the child's regression to earlier psychosexual stages (e.g., wanting to be carried to bed, sexually stimulating other children, making or cleaning up messes). Often children wish to become very "groupy" to avoid the task of reducing stimuli from the external world; therefore, much of the management is individualized and teaches children to look inward a little (emphasis on snacks, pleasant anticipations of the next day). Deviations can be handled by teaching the child about the ineffectiveness of his defense, or by suggesting some alternative behavior. Such teaching tends to be more of an insight experience, although much learning by imitation also occurs.

An especially helpful management action at this point is breaking the next step in the routine into small pieces that children can follow. Instead of asking the children to get ready for showers, the child-care worker might need only to ask them to go to their bedroom, and, when this is done, to get undressed. This segmenting of the routine externalizes some of the ego's "programming" of events. It tends to limit the magnitude of the child's anxiety and limits the issue of his fight if he makes one. It decreases the possibilities for large-scale acting-out and enables the children to feel more comfortable and secure.

Undressing and showering

Once the children are in the bedroom-shower area, their task is to get undressed and take showers. There are many possibilities for ego failure at this step. Fears of undressing in front of others, overstimulation in undressing and in seeing other children undressed, and fears of exposure and bodily injury are common. The child-care worker can help by assuring privacy or being assuring about bodily integrity, or simply by getting the child started in the routine by untying his shoes or pulling off his boots.

Which pair of children shower at the same time (we have two separate but "equal" showers) is known, and does not vary (except if children shower early). Children have towels (passed out to them before they come to the shower) or wear bathrobes to avoid exposing themselves. They learn to use the conventions of modesty as an ego skill. The male child-care worker adjusts the shower before the child gets in (to prevent scalding or a sudden dowsing with cold water, and to show that an adult is in charge) and sees that there are soap and a face cloth. He reminds the child to wash various parts of his body. As showers become more and more pleasurable, children want to shower for longer periods and bring more toys with them.

Not only do we protect children from certain kinds of stimulation when they are undressing, showering, and drying off, but we also design our verbal messages to fit the process of going to sleep. Learning how to care for, protect, and manage one's body helps the child to master some of the fear associated with his body. It is this kind of alternate behavior that has the greatest potential for enabling the child to cope with this part of the bedtime situation.

Such teaching necessitates rather close supervision of the children and close communication among the managing adults. The adults must tell each other where the children are in the routine and whether a particular child has a special problem or a special need. Because the routine must remain flexible enough to accommodate the specific needs of the children, communication among the adults must be open and continuous.

Between showers and "lights out"

When the child comes out of the shower and is ready to go to his room, he must be "picked up" by the other child-care worker (usually female), who sees that the child gets into pajamas and has something to do until the lights are put out. This is a good time to talk over events of the day and the coming events of tomorrow, to anticipate the next morning with the early riser, to give some support to the child and allay the fears that he expresses. It is easier to handle potential upsets at this point than after the lights are out, when other children are trying to go to sleep. In general, children are more susceptible to "contagion" after the lights are out. Fear is often sharper when the child feels more alone.

This is a crucial point in the routine. The managing adults have helped the child to switch from daytime activities to preparation for sleep and tried to focus his attention on the care of his body as a part of the larger process of going from wakefulness to sleep. Their conversations have attempted to facilitate dealing with internal stimuli by verbalizing them. Teaching children to cope with fears in this way is possible because it is structured into the routine and is based upon knowledge of the ego processes necessary for getting to sleep.

Getting into bed, lights out, snacks

After showers are over, the child-care worker picks up dirty clothes, hands out clothes for the next day, giving the child a limited choice in some part of his wardrobe (e.g., color of socks), and puts the clothes where the child wants them for the morning. In general, the adult should honor requests to get things if they are within reason. All this basically reassures the child that there will be a tomorrow, that we are concerned about his appearance, and that we will help him arrange his world in a comfortable and protective way (many requests are about adjusting window shades, lights, doors, extra blankets, and Band-aids).

The child-care worker then urges and assists the child into bed. When a room is reasonably settled, lights are turned off and snacks are given out. This snack is timed as a reward for ego-based accomplishment. It takes advantage of the child's body concerns and channels them into the pleasurable experience of eating. The child-care worker (usually female) says good night to the children and sees that they are comfortable. The style of saying good night varies from child to child. Some like to be tucked in and wish to go to sleep immediately;

others wait until they are more settled, then ask a child-care worker to do something for them; some wish to go to the bathroom or to get a drink of water.

After the "goodnight rounds" are completed, the child-care worker (usually male) sits in a central hall and reads a story to the entire group.[3] We select stories with care, using such criteria as intelligibility, interest, and whether they produce fear. From the hall, the child-care worker can also offer reassurance, answer questions for an individual child, and, at the same time, speak to the unspoken worries of other children. After about twenty or thirty minutes of reading (when most of the children are asleep), the child-care worker shuts off the main lights in the hall and remains there until all the children are asleep. Some lights are left on so that children can find their way to the bathroom. There is also a small night light in each bedroom.

The child becomes most aware of internal stimuli when the lights have been turned out and he is lying in his bed. Our routine has been designed to manage this heightened awareness of internal stimuli. Snacks and stories not only pleasantly tone these stimuli, but also provide reassurance through the presence of adults. Nevertheless, there are frequently times when these management techniques do not meet the needs of the child sufficiently. In this context, however, it becomes easier for the child to state his fears and thereby to learn appropriate coping mechanisms.

In answer to mild fear, we tell the child which adult will be present during the night, which child-care worker will come in the morning, who lives on grounds, and about the existence of lightning rods (during storms) and the strength of the house. For a "day-residue" problem, we tell the child that he can see the appropriate person the next day. If acting out or bizarre behavior continues, we tell the child that he cannot keep others awake. Sometimes the presence of an adult in a bedroom enables the child to relax and sleep. Sitting close to

[3] We have a bedroom area consisting of three bedrooms, a small "quiet" room, and a bathroom, all of which branch off a central hall. There are two three-child rooms, and one two-child room. Each child has his own area, with a bed, shelves, bureau, bulletin board, and a night stand.

an adult, or in a lighted room, gives the very frightened child a sense of protection. Removal from the bedroom to a lighted single bedroom near the story-reader is most often used when a child begins to "infect" other children in the room. Return to the room is dependent on the climate of the room and the ability of the removed child to manage the task of going to sleep. Child-care workers try to be rather non-verbal at later times of the night by enforcing quiet, whispering, and avoiding conversations, using stock answers to the more outlandish questions.

The gross behavior deviations that would tend to destroy a routine are managed within a broader context. Methods of dealing with a highly agitated child or a very depressed child can be worked out beforehand so that managing their behavior can be routinized. We have used early bedtimes with little success, and have found that short afternoon naps are more helpful. The nap seems to provide an opportunity for the child to practice coping with the ego tasks of bedtime alone with the child-care worker. It is unusual for the child actually to fall asleep at this time; rather, there is much discussion of the individual issues and affects involved in the bedtime routine.

We do not guarantee that our routine, or any routine, will produce "smooth," trouble-free bedtimes in institutions for children. Our procedure does, however, tend to insure that bedtime will be managed in a manner consistent with the treatment of the child. It keeps the handling of the events at bedtime within the context of teaching adaptive behavior to the child.

VII
UNDERSTANDING THE STAGES OF A TYPICAL TEMPER TANTRUM

Albert E. Trieschman

The cursing, fighting, wild anger of a child is an alarming sight to the adult in charge of him. The destructiveness of a temper tantrum not only frightens adults but demands that protective actions be taken by them. Being forced to take action and being at least mildly frightened are a troublesome combination. It is the kind of situation that produces many inappropriate ideas and non-therapeutic actions—ranging from gross oversimplifications of what is going on, to actual counterattacks on the child. This chapter is an effort to helpfully complicate the view of a temper tantrum by presenting it as a series of ego conditions. It is largely based on observations of borderline psychotic and character disordered boys (7–12 years of age) in residential treatment at Walker Home. We will analyze the sequence of events that characterize the apparently sudden "falling apart" of the child's usual functioning called a tantrum. We will gear our description to both understanding and managing the episode. Our focus is on the events of the tantrum itself, those immediately preceding it, and those following soon afterwards. We are not dismissing the importance of a child's life history in understanding tantrums, nor are we dismissing the knowledge that mismanagement by adults sometimes provokes tantrums. We simply have not found that examination of these variables gives a very complete understanding of the immediate events of the tantrum, and have found them even less helpful to managing the tantrum as it occurs. Our effort is to supplement not supplant the individual psychogenetics of tantrums.

We have found that it is quite impossible to prevent many of the temper tantrums among our seriously disturbed 7- to 12-year-olds. Skillful efforts at planning interesting activities and well-arranged daily routines certainly do help to reduce tantrums. It is the idle boring unprogrammed hours that promote impulse-ridden naughtiness among children in residential treatment programs. The boredom often comes to mean lack of safety and security to the child just because the children's impulses begin to program the time—and their impulses often frighten them. Interrupting this naughtiness does set off some tantrums. Carefully dealing with staff feelings about children can reduce the occasions that adults "unconsciously provoke" temper tantrums. But despite good programs and minimal provocation by adults, disturbed children in superior treatment programs have tantrums. Why? We think the answer is simply that emotionally disturbed children often behave like younger children, like young children in the midst of trying to work out a self image or struggling to balance their dependence on others with their desire to be more independent. It is, of course, at just this phase of development (typically 2 to 3 years of age) that tantrums are considered "normal" (Stone and Church, 1957, pp. 112–113). It is also our belief that children engaged in treatment programs are struggling to change their maladaptive behavior—and that this struggle is a disquieting one. Giving up old ways (symptoms) and learning new growth skills often leaves the child uncomfortably between old and new. Sometimes his only resource for filling this gap in the process of growth and change is a loud, disturbing, even dangerous act of desperation like a tantrum. In short, temper tantrums are to be expected in residential treatment facilities. And staff need not assume the guilty burden that all tantrums occur out of program failure or staff inadequacy or, worse, that some adult unconsciously provoked the child to the wild attack. There is no doubt that there is much to be learned about programs or routines from observing the timing of upsets. We simply must not assume that we can chase away the phenomena of tantrums with a "perfected program" and a "purified unconscious."

The remainder of this chapter is divided into three sections: (1) a brief examination of some clichéd attitudes and handling advice about tantrums, concluding with our schema of the ego mechanisms involved in the kind of tantrums we are describing; (2) a detailed look at the six stages we have observed in most temper tantrums including general management advice for each stage; and (3) a concluding section which summarizes the stage theory and draws some implications.

Bad Advice and Incomplete Theory

The awesome sight of the tantrum's pounding, flailing, shouting energy demands a sane understanding word from the adult experienced with children. And the advice is forthcoming. However, about the only aspect the various statements have in common is the certainty with which they are spoken:

> "He just wants attention." . . . "Put him in a room by himself where he can't get hurt." . . . "Walk away and remove the audience." . . . "I find if you just laugh at the ridiculous waste of energy, it will stop." . . . "Any kid who shows he wants to fight me will find out I'm bigger and tougher." . . . "If he thinks he can get his way with that act, he better think again." . . . "The poor child is frightened—comfort him and hold him close."

Each of these statements contains the customary "grain of truth." Power struggle, attention-getting device, episode of childhood terror, energy discharge, psychotic-like rage, disassociated affect state—these are the more technical terms that one hears about temper tantrums. And, as we will see, each of the terms and each of the statements describes some part of the tantrum or its meaning to the child. But most of the advice tends to be very partial and the implication is that the tantrum is composed of a single event or a series of identical events. If that were so, perhaps a single explanation or antidote would suffice, but it is not so. The typical temper tantrum is described more accurately as a developing series of events, periods of which have different characteristics. It is because the behavior that composes most of the tantrum is sufficiently offensive or frightening that we easily lump it together as one terrible event (for us and for the child). We come to fix in our minds oversimplified versions of what happened, disguised moral stances about how bad they are, or guilt relief about how harmless they are. Then we fix some quickie cure like "isolate him" and try to forget those poignant yet painful (often to our ribs) moments that we live through periodically.

In order that there be no confusion about what events we consider tantrums, let us eliminate what is not included. Group hell-raising, wild as it sometimes gets, is not considered a bunch of temper tantrums. I do not believe I have ever seen more than one real temper tantrum going on at the same time. It is possible that the other children within view recognize the anguish involved and damp down their own inclinations to cry out to the adults for help. My observation is that the children standing around are awestruck by the struggle and very careful to note what the adult is feeling and doing. Temper tantrums should not be confused with quiet solitary acts of destruction or with a wild fight between children. Nor are we including an ordinary argument with a child. These events have some aspects in common with tantrums but require other understanding and management. Redl and Wineman deal with such topics in their work on Pioneer House (1950). We are referring only to those loud, rather public (with at least an adult around), angry, uncontrolled episodes of impulse discharged by a single child. They are frequent enough in any residential treatment program that no one can be very long in doubt about having seen one.

Some notions about the ego form the basis of our stage theory of tantrums. The psychoanalytic version of anxiety and ego functioning is our base.

We need some ego theory in order to get on to the stages of the tantrum. A modified psychoanalytic version of anxiety and ego functioning will serve us well (Freud, 1949, pp. 109–

112). Anxiety—a feeling of anticipated discomfort or dread —functions in the organized ego as a danger signal. It warns the ego of some inner impulse danger, or some outer real threat, or of some sense of impending helplessness. It signals the ego to call into play defenses and coping skills. The ego's success lies in its capacity to modify and guide thoughts and actions in the direction of satisfaction and safety. We should add that the ego's success also depends on its capacity to see its thoughts and actions affecting the world of things and people. That view gives the child his sense of self-esteem and competence (White, 1963, pp. 33–43).

The young child of 2 or 3 does not have a very organized, richly defended ego for avoiding discomfort, nor is his backlog of competence and self-esteem sufficient to feel no sense of helplessness and incompetence. It is similar with our character-disordered, ego-damaged patients of 7 to 12. They clearly feel anxiety and discomfort but its signal is often not very clear—more akin to suppressed panic than signal anxiety. Moreover, their defenses and coping skills are often primitive and irratic. Add to that the likelihood in the therapeutic residence that the child is uncomfortably between old reactions and new skills, and you have an ego often on the verge of being overwhelmed with a sense of helplessness.

It is our view that the temper tantrum can be profitably seen as a series of efforts on the part of the child's ego to signal his sense of danger and helplessness, to seek help, and, at the same time, to maintain a semblance of the feeling that he can still effect his world through his own efforts. We think we can demonstrate that the wild disruption of the tantrum is a primitive last ditch effort to maintain the ego's sense of self-esteem. The series of events composing the tantrum encompass the deterioration of the ego as well as the ego's efforts to forestall and then compensate for the deterioration. This brief statement is barely what we need to understand the stages of a tantrum. It should not be taken as a complete ego theory. If it hints that our point of view leans toward the importance of mastery of the environment as an essential and non-instinctual aspect of the ego, we have revealed our bias.

Typical Stages of a Temper Tantrum

The stages of the temper tantrum are intended as descriptions of the child's effort to maintain control and self-esteem in the face of ego deterioration. We think of the stages as an ordered sequence of predominant themes in behavior as the tantrum progresses. No two tantrums, even by the same child, are identical. All of us can call to mind many varieties of noises and actions in a tantrum. As each stage is described, we will give some attention to its *various appearances in behavior.* At each stage, we will deal in some detail with what the child is feeling and what he seems to be trying to accomplish. We have called that the *inner dynamics* of the stage. Because *therapeutic management* is a primary concern, we also will discuss what we would like to help the child learn at each stage. What actions we can take, what arrangements we can make, even what helpful things might be said will be mentioned. Of course, the child-care worker's or therapist's relationship with the child, his experience, and his ingenuity can often upstage us here. Perhaps we can promote some new ingenuity and save some old relationships with difficult children. Our view is that the tantrum is an inefficient means of coping with feelings and reality. Our goal is to understand its immediate process sufficiently well to teach the child alternative coping behavior to survive his ego crises. The alternatives that we help the child learn are better matches to reality than a tantrum, and they are more likely to salvage a sense of competence and self-esteem for the child. Our single mindedness about the tantrums immediate events and on-the-spot adult interventions is not intended, of course, as a substitute for all our other therapeutic work with the child.

Our stages are named for the characteristic behavior sequence we have noted in a tantrum: (1) Rumbling and Grumbling, (2) Help-Help, (3) Either-Or, (4) No-No, (5) Leave Me Alone, and (6) Hangover.

In going right through all six stages—and the description, dynamics, and management for each—we do not imply that a tantrum inevitably runs this whole course, and we especially do not imply that no relationship or skillful management ever stops a tantrum short of its full course. The stages are a conceptual framework around which to organize observation, speculation, and management of a particular child's tantrum—hopefully in a more discriminating way than our present global labels and quickie cures. Because they are intended to function as a conceptual framework, we have included the possible entire sequence of events in the tantrum.

Rumbling and Grumbling

In this first stage, the child walks around the grounds of the treatment center or perhaps "knocks around" in the cottage. He looks grouchy. He grumbles grudging hellos to a passersby. He scowls. Often he is dribbling (as opposed to gushing) hostility. For example, he quietly marks up a chair he is sitting on or he whacks at trees or railings he passes. Occasionally, he makes an attempt at silly comic relief, briefly giggling about something. He looks uncomfortable in his own skin. Nothing really seems to satisfy him; he complains about what is offered, but seems equally dissatisfied with his own choices. Something is brewing. He eyes the action around him, makes forays toward it, but rarely joins except briefly. He seems to be fighting himself, the child-care worker, and especially the growing panic within himself. Sooner or later, he develops an issue to which he can attach importance. He has settled on a time and place. Some children have characteristic issues or characteristic times and places. For others, a pattern in this visible sense is difficult to determine.

Tom usually "discovered" some loss. "Whatever happened to that little red car I had?" He would remember in great detail where he bought it, how unique it was, how you failed to take care of it despite its obvious "great importance" to him. You have wronged him greatly, and you cannot even remember the car.

Joe actually appeared to search for a broken toy. For example, he would examine a piece of a model airplane wing to determine if it could be from his model of long ago. Once he discovered a broken possession, he ran to demand its repair by the child-care worker.

Will would carefully lay the groundwork to be scapegoated. He would tell boys family information, say he did not want anyone to know, and then aggravate a tormentor until the information was shouted back at him. He would then have his issue: "You don't care that they pick on me."

Don, for a long time, had tantrums or near-tantrums right before a trip. The anticipation of a trip, in fact, seemed to start him rumbling and grumbling.

Inner Dynamics. The rumbling and grumbling seems to be the child's effort to manage his vague internal sense of discomfort, growing helplessness, and even near panic. His own anxiety is too vague and in itself dangerously close to overwhelming to serve as a signal to mobilize ego-maintaining defenses. The defenses themselves are either in flux or inadequate for the strong feelings he has. And so he seeks a concrete external issue, time, and place to represent his vague feelings—something to "get his teeth into." Occasionally the issue picked is representative of feelings that are especially overwhelming to that particular child: Tom's deep sense of loss, Joe's broken family, Will's chronic sense of being different and worse than any boy ever was. Sometimes, the time and place (for example, bedtime, mealtime, a trip in a car) are representative of an especially troublesome (or even traumatic) event or set of feelings. Often the issue picked is peculiarly unresolvable: the broken toy is clearly not able to be repaired, the time chosen makes individual attention nearly impossible, the long-lost item is clearly not recoverable. From the child-care worker's point of view, it looks just like the issue and time and place are chosen by the child just *because* resolution through adult helpfulness is so difficult. Perhaps the choice is no accident. The inner dynamic task of the ego is a horrendous one—and probably needs a horrendous external effort on the part of the child-care worker to help the child carry out his ego repair. The external "staging" of the tantrum with its difficult timing and apparently unresolvable issue is an "accurate" externalization of the internal ego drama.

Management Suggestions. Careful observations of the child are the crucial aspect of management in this first stage. Over time, they give us knowledge about his particular vulnerabilities and about his characteristic issues, times, and places. We can begin to distinguish long-term rumblers from abbreviated rumblers, loud open grumblers from more quiet, less visible ones. Once we can see what is going on, we can often help the child package his issue in a more manageable size. We can help him to verbalize his growing discomfort.

With Bill, it was often possible to recall a long list of times that his mood was represented by looking for something that could be called "lost forever." He began to be able to use his own behavior as a signal to himself, a signal that he was feeling rotten (thrown away and lost). With this verbal translation, he could often engage a child-care worker in a conversation directed at basic restitution of his own sense of worth.

In the early phases of treatment this often does precious little and may even be a provocation. Of course, it is extremely easy to be "the straw that broke the ego's back" when a child is rumbling. We all feel guilty when we see ourselves trigger a tantrum issue with a direction or comment we make. In work with ego-defective children, this is often unavoidable. Moreover, the prolonged grumble and rumble is debilitating to the child's participation in the fun, activities, and routines of the residence. In fact, there are times when getting the tantrum "over with" is helpful to the child and the situation. It can have an "air-clearing" quality, especially if the child-care worker has a strong relationship with the youngster and can attenuate the tantrum. Other times dictate that a child-care worker relationship (especially one that is going to be needed in the next hours for a trip) should be protected. In that situation, it is often wise to have another child-care worker engage the child on the tantrum issue. A power figure in the milieu—director, chief child-care worker—can often damp down a tantrum in its initial stage, an effect than can also be produced by the appearance of a stranger. A switch in child-care workers handling the child can also pacify the engagement—but it should be remembered that one does not always want to "prevent" or postpone a tantrum. Once the child has settled on an issue, a time, and a place, the rumble and grumble quickly builds to louder, more anguished noises.

Help-Help

This next stage of the tantrum begins the real noisy engagement. The child has realized his wish to externalize his ego struggle. He has found the issue and is now signaling his need for help. The signal he uses is usually a very visible and deliberate rule-breaking act—an iconoclastic roar of some sort. Its form is dependent on what the child knows about the institution's sacred cows and what his particular problems are. He may curse loudly and vilely; he may throw something at the child-care worker; he may attack another child or get himself attacked; he may break something; he may expose his genitals—in short, he pointedly violates some generally accepted canon of behavior. He pushes one of the system's panic buttons—i.e., he does something that he knows will alarm the child-care worker. He "gives us his panic" in order to call "Help-Help." Let there be no doubt, if we had no rules or sacred cows or codes of our own, the child would find some "Help-Help" call that demanded the immediate intervention of an adult. The noise and activity of the panic button should, and usually does, cause the adult to move very close to the child in order to stop the forbidden act. At this point, the child-care worker often has to hold the child physically for the sake of his own and the child's safety. However, some youngsters (e.g., more passive character disorders) thrash about fairly safely and only require the closeness of the adult who has heard their signal (and responded by stopping the rule breach). Other youngsters require holding only in the next stage of the tantrum when they are threatening more violence. At this juncture, the child is feeling his own incapacity to hold back his impulses and his signal demands that the adult's hands, voice, and closeness provide him some limitation, some external control. A child-care worker needs to assure the safety that the child no longer feels he can provide for himself. His overwhelming anger frightens him; his behavior signals his need for control and help.

Inner Dynamics. We have anticipated some of the feelings of the child in the description of this stage. The parallel between the effect of the child's attention-getting, forbidden act on an adult and the operation of signal anxiety on an organized ego seems to me quite informative. The child's "Help-Help" behavior operates to bring a restraining influence (an adult) into the picture in analogy to the manner in which signal anxiety mobilizes defenses against impulses. The disturbed child (or the young child) carries out interpersonally what more normal or mature ego functioning carries out "intra-personally." It only remains to detail the ways in which the restraining adult can become a helpful protective "ego" for the "tantrumming" child. Hopefully, the child-care worker can manage the child in such a way that he models (teaches) more mature ego-based coping skills than the child's screaming violent behavior. One easily overlooked aspect of this stage is the child's tremendous feeling of defeat. His impulsive outburst brings with it a sense of failure ("I've done that bad thing again") and visible evidence (the adult) that he cannot control himself. Of course, this is the reason that the child-care worker's prompt answer to the "Help-Help" signal is not welcomed with open arms and a "thank you." The child's rage at ego disintegration is turned on the adult. Even in that rage, however, there seems to be an attempt by the child to salvage a sense of self. We will describe our version of that compensatory effort as we discuss the later stages of the tantrum.

Management Suggestions. The description of behavior and the hypothetical inner dynamics we have given suggest the management a child-care worker needs to carry out at the "Help-Help" stage. He needs to provide the control the child is "out of" and to do this in a way conducive to teaching the child some alternative signaling and behavior controlling skills. A realistic caution: Do not expect that management at this point can be a calm insight-promoting psychotherapy session. The wild child struggling in your arms does not have enough ego to control his own body, much less enough ego to attend to any subtle comments on your part about his past, his parents, or his problems. Do not hesitate to give your directions to him loudly, clearly, and repetitively. Hold him no more firmly than is necessary (and from behind so that neither of you gets hurt). Your body (controlled by your ego) holds his body which he cannot hold. Avoid the temptation to squeeze him tightly out of your anger. Tell him what you are doing:

"You can't keep your body from hurting yourself and others. I am going to hold you until you can control it again. [Child lunges to bite.] No. I am not going to let you hurt me and I will try to keep you from hurting yourself. . . . [Child: You're trying to kill me!] No—this is not a fight; I am trying *not* to hurt you. Your struggling is dangerous. I can let you go only when you can control your body. [I have seen experienced child-care workers actually return a limb at a time to the child's control.]

The aim of the child-care worker is to assure control and safety. He needs to verbalize that the child's behavior demands the holding operation. Phrases like "S.O.S." "Help-Help" can sometimes be given to the child in order to communicate the idea of signaling. Saying "You have that 'throw something,' 'break something' feeling" can help to establish your point: i.e., that the child has some feelings he is trying to defend against.

Bob raced into the dining room and wildly knocked over chairs. I got him as he was shoving the table over. As I put my arms around him, I naïvely asked, "How do you feel?" He shouted, "Nothin', nothin'. You idiot, I don't feel nothin'."

Later, he said that when he raced around and knocked over things, he was unable to feel anything (anger, sadness, etc.). He acknowledged that feeling "nothin'" was a desirable state—and one of the reasons he acted wildly when he was desperate.

The meaningful establishment of some recognizable warning feelings inside him really has to wait until later in the child's tantrum. The most that can be accomplished at this point is control, safety, and a blunt message about feelings. Later, we need to go over what in the child's behavior signaled to us and help him establish some awareness for himself of a safer signal.

With many children, some bodily sensation—clenching fists, stomach pain, a desire to run—can be established in their consciousness as a safer signal than the wild behavior they used to signal the adult.

A few other suggestions about management of this stage apply generally enough to warrant mentioning. If holding can be safely avoided or postponed, do so. If the child's impulsive signaling behavior is to dash to some high place (up a tree, on the top of some climbing apparatus), do not chase up after him as they do in those dramatic endings of gangster movies. You will probably decrease safety in the situation if you do. You can be reasonably close, protective, and in fair control of the situation by talking to him from below. Another obvious suggestion is: do not get in some refined legalistic argument about "you know the rules about climbing trees or breaking windows or throwing things." He probably does know the rules and his "Help-Help" behavior was chosen because of the rule. Whenever possible get him to some comfortable, unpublic place—perhaps a bed or a couch.

Some children, during what we are calling the "Help-Help" stage attempt to get the child-care worker to play externally a role similar to the one played internally by the primitive superego. They demand to know the consequences or punishment for their bad behavior. Their insistence on a sin and penance system may be difficult to avoid, but it should be avoided. It has seemed to us that the child is "baiting" the adult into punishing him as if he could substitute a harsh punishment for an ego defense. Whether the milieu has a network of punishments (automatic negative consequences for particular misbehavior, e.g., restrictions of privileges, demerits, etc.), it is important not to let the affirmation of or argumentation about punishment become the focus of your conversation with the child. If you do, your are agreeing that penance or punishment is a substitute for ego modulation of behavior in the out-of-control situation. And, of course, much acting out is just such an operation, i.e., the "misdeed" is a self-punishing act unconsciously intended as penance for an original sin. Of course, the repentance is often more destructive than the sin. Later you may need or want to employ some "punishment" (restriction, separation from group) for reasons of group hygiene (*à* la Redl) or as a means of helping "shut down" a child's guilt over misbehavior. Affirming or arguing some later punishment with a child, however, is not to be substituted for firm limit setting in the upset situation itself.

Either-Or

In this stage the major theme of the child's behavior is a combination of impossible alternatives, threats and demands. The child-care worker is likely to be still holding the child, or at least in close control. From that range the child shouts his wishes.

> Either you let me kill him or I'll kill you. . . . Find my car or I'll break a window. . . . I'm gonna get a machine gun and kill everybody. . . . Let me go so I can smash him. . . . If you hold me forever, I'll still kill him [even though he had gotten himself attacked by another larger stronger child]. . . . Fix my plane now or I'll smash it. . . . You stole my thing and I'm gonna steal something of yours.

Words of primitive vengeance, grandiose brutality, and ugly omnipotence—shouted or gritted-teeth versions of these stream from the child. As an added component, the child is often personally abusive to the adult. He ridicules (often sexually) some characteristic of the adult's body or personality. It is noteworthy that the child is often extremely discriminating about which barbs are effective. In the midst of apparently complete loss of control, the child may still be sensitive to fairly subtle interpersonal signs that he has "got to the adult." Of course, he then repeats that particular abuse mercilessly.

> "You're fat, or dumb." . . . Confused sexual disparagements, or accusations of sexual liasons with familiar adults are common, as are taunting sexual invitations.

Inner Dynamics. Paradoxically we see in these threats, insults, and impossible alternatives the struggle of the child's ego to hold on to some shred of self, some sense of competence or at least efficacy. He is screaming his necessity to feel that he has some options left. He seems to be demanding that reality yield to his efforts to manipulate it. This observation suggests that even in the midst of this impulsive and instinctual flood, the child's need for some efficacy exists. It hints that the ego, even when awash in the impulsive flood of the tantrum, contains an aspect that struggles to affect the environment. It adds credence to the existence, within the ego, of an independent, non-instinctual "effectance behavior" which White has formalized (1963). In simpler terms, the child has been robbed of feelings of bodily control, but he continues to propose action alternatives (even ridiculous ones) as though options were the essence of self. The struggle to affect the feelings of the adult (the insults) is only one version of the child's "crash program" for affecting the environment of people and things. His "Either-Or" and "threatening" words are an omnipotent assimilation of casuality to himself. The tantruming child temporarily becomes a Frankenstein-like version of Piaget's scientist-child. What we are stressing here is that through all the threatening noise, one can often hear the compensatory efforts of the ego. The child attempts to compensate for his loss of control by exaggerating his sense of manipulating the environment. The very impulses that are overwhelming him are loosely packaged as tools for making some kind of effect on the environment. What effect seems less crucial than that the child see himself as the cause of effects. (Some readers will note that much of the behavior and dynamics of this stage could be described in psychoanalytic terms as breakthrough of feelings of omnipotence in the face of the crumbled ego.)

Management Suggestions. By this stage of the tantrum, tempers are high. Some adults are mistakenly drawn into argument over the insults, threats, and impossible alternatives. They methodically try to rebut the child's proposals but soon are caught in a web of contradictions and subject changes. Exasperation joins the debate. The child gets some pleasure from the adult's tormented struggle to maintain logic and consistency. Vindictive aggression toward the child is very tempting. Other adults become very uncomfortable with their own rising anger and take an overly passive attitude: "Sticks and stones will break my bones but names will never hurt me." The adult's sullen protest to the child that "you can't make me angry" is unrealistic. It often functions as an invitation to the child to escalate his behavior. The situation appears so boundless to the child that he becomes more agitated—and more desperate. Time and space boundaries seem to loosen in the child's mind and he begins to extend his vendetta beyond the "here and now."

> I'm gonna get a gun and kill you. . . . When I'm 21, you better watch out. . . .

Maintaining time and place boundaries for the child is extremely important in this stage of the tantrum.

> You and I are staying right here. . . . I am going to hold you until you can hold yourself. . . . We'll get this all straightened out by supper time [some time dimension the child knows]. . . . This won't last forever. . . .

Any "Either-Or" proposal that is sensible or can be shifted toward a legitimate sequence of events should be accepted and promoted. Occasionally, the adult can modify a child's ridiculous proposal—"either fix it or I smash it"—to a reasonable one—"either we can try to fix it or we can replace the model." Seeking alternatives in an attempt to feel you have control over a situation is a reasonable coping skill that we would hope to teach children. Often no such opportunity appears. Then we have to insist that the child's impossible alternatives, threats, and insults are not the only way to effect the situation.

> That may be the only choice you have, but there are other things to do. I can give you some other choices to make.
>
> or
>
> Those are *your* only choices. That is all you can think you can do. But I have other choices. I am going to stay with you until this is over and then we will find a better way to get this settled.

In the second example above the adult is not really giving the child other choices but modeling that human beings have choices even when they are "uptight."

Another helpful adult reaction at this stage of the tantrum is modeling a reasonable expression of anger. Tell a child that you are angry at what he is doing, that you do not like what he is doing, sounding and looking angry as you say this. Helpfully modeling reasonable anger is something a child could imitate more easily than boundless patience and complete impassivity in the face of fury.

If seeking legitimate "Either-Ors," broadening alternatives bounding the situation in time and place, and modeling reasonable anger all fail to stem the tantrum, it proceeds to the next stage—a further ego entrenchment.

No-No

As the threats and impossible alternatives are denied reality by the adult and no reasonable alternative is found, the child often retreats into a more primitive version of self. He makes it clear that, although he cannot take action, he is not doing what you ask. He tends to decrease his positive attempts to effect events and increase his negations (in word and deed) of your words and actions.

If you pull his arm slightly in one direction, he pulls the other direction. If you say lie comfortably, he trys to get up or vice versa. If you offer to help him out of his jacket, he pulls it around himself.

The major theme of this stage is the child's denial or negation of adult ideas, comments, or directions. Although he may have done some negating earlier, the behavior at this stage is most exclusively based on negations. While earlier the child was mainly proposing and the adult mainly disposing, the child is now mainly disposing of what the adult is proposing.

"Don't talk to me." . . . "Shut up!" . . . "Don't touch my bed, my toy." . . . If the adult suggests quiet or calm, the child yells or produces a flurry of movements. If the adult talks about help, the child twists his body to promote hurt.

The negations, denials and reversals of this stage have an almost obsessive and automatic quality.

Inner Dynamics. We think of the negativism of the "No-No" stage as a primitive ego defense of identity. The child's inability to hold onto his identity as a cause of effects ("Either-Or" stage) is followed by a retreat to a simpler identity. In effect, he is saying, "I can't cause any action but I am me because I am not you." *Me* is defined as "not you or your wishes for me." The effect of the overwhelming impulse flood of the tantrum is to primitivize the ego. But what is very clear is that the child continues struggling to maintain some identity. The dynamic of the "No-No" is thought of as the last interpersonal defense of the sense of self.

It is interesting to compare the role of negation as a primitive defense of identity and as a process involved in the origin of a sense of identity. The early "No-No's" of the toddler are usually in the service of autonomy striving. The testing of the power of self is carried out through negations of the wishes of the parent. In the absence of one's own proposals for action, one negates another person's proposals in order to feel some sense of competence and control of events. It seems quite natural that a process that is one of the foundations of the self should be relied on later in life at times when the remainder of self-structure has crumbled, as in the tantrum.

Management Suggestions. The rudimentary ego that remains by this stage of the tantrum makes it difficult to deal with the child. The values that adults hold dear are easily chewed up by the negations of the child. This stage is not a good time to tell the child how much you want to *help* him ("You want to kill me"), how much you still like him ("You hate me"), or how he will feel better soon ("I'm never gonna stop hating you"). Feeding the child the philosophy of the institution—the system's goals and values about getting help, getting well—is predictably going to produce denials and reversals.

About the safest position for the adult to take is one premised on the desire for the child to regain more self and more self control.

I want you to be your own boss again. . . . You can be in charge of yourself when you can say "No" to all this silliness, craziness, thrashing around, etc.

The shifting of some of the negation to denying energy to the thrashing limbs works "miraculously"—when it works, which is only occasionally. Helping the child to see the infantile quality of the "No-No" self can sometimes be promoted by a "yes-no" game or directions by opposites. The automatic way in which the child does the opposite of what you ask (or negates what you say) can sometimes produce a humorous breakthrough. Suddenly the child "sees" the silliness of the whole thing when he finds himself saying or doing what you want him to because you "cleverly" stated the opposite of what you really wanted. This is a tricky gimmick to try. It depends on an old relationship with the child, a gentle sense of humor, and the child's having some remaining observing ego to see the humor. If these conditions do not apply, do not try this. The resulting humiliation and derogation to the child will be far more damaging than any little piece of cooperation you cleverly get.

If some rudimentary sense of self-control develops at this stage, it is often possible to push the tantrum back to the alternative proposing stage ("Either-Or") and begin to develop some reasonable actions or "if-then" sequences with the child. If no comfortable ego control develops during the "No-No" stage, the tantrum gradually runs down. The struggling diminishes and depression begins to replace aggression. The struggling ego retreats from the interpersonal sphere and draws inward.

Leave Me Alone

Gradually the movement and talk of the child become more perfunctory. Though occasional bursts of negativism appear, the child seems more placid or sad. He may allow you to help him to get into a more comfortable position or tolerate your help in removing a jacket or adjusting a pillow or cushion. Crying and yelling or taunting are replaced by a rather hollow, distant-sounding voice. Manneristic mouth movements are frequent—pursing or sucking in lips, licking or biting the lips. The child often checks over his body—feeling his arm or leg, wiping his eyes, adjusting an article of clothing. The adult who has stayed with the child has a peaceful moment and begins to notice the red face and red eyes of a tired child. An offer of water and a cool cloth may be accepted.

The verbalizations of the child, and his movements, suggest his desire to avoid, or at least curtail, interaction with the adult. He does not look at you, buries his head under covers, pulls his shirt over his eyes, blocks his ears, occasionally even gets under a bed or in a closet. His acceptance of your help (water, getting comfortable) is brief and is clearly not intended to re-establish a warm friendly conversation (and should not be exploited for this purpose by the adult). Your attempts at engagement with the child will usually be rebuffed.

Leave me alone. . . . Don't talk to me. . . . Get out of here. . . . Don't bug me. . . . Don't look at me. . . .

A mixture of relative calm, sadness and a desire to minimize interaction seem to characterize this stage.

Inner Dynamics. The ego's inability to maintain identity or a sense of competence even through negations of the adult's directions ("No-No" stage) produces a considerable defeat. The result is a withdrawal of engagement or fight with the outside world and amounts to brief depression. A smaller solipstic *me* (all alone and directed inward) is temporarily all that remains for the ego to defend. It does so by ceasing to interact with the outside world. Licking wounds and incapsulating this self serve to direct energy inward where they are needed. It seems as though the depression functions adaptively to "cut back" on the behavior directed toward the world.

The relative calm of this stage can be mistaken for the "return of the ego." Because the child is no longer a wild, fighting creature, adults sometimes conclude that he is back in control. They try to rejoin him in ordinary interaction or they quickly put him back into the stream of daily events. The suddenness with which the child "falls apart" again is testimony to his ego's fragility. Depression, especially in acting-out children, can look a little like ego functioning. Nothing terrible is happening, to be sure, but that is because so little of anything is coming out of the child. Depression, in this case, is a "fake ego."

Management Suggestions. It is important to respect the child's withdrawal during this stage. Some adults are tempted to launch into a lecture on the foolishness or dangers of temper tantrums. Don't. It is usually sensible to allow the child to block out external stimuli—under his covers, blocking his ears—as a means of protecting his fragile "me-alone" ego state. Not looking at the child or moving away a little can be a helpful means of respecting his wish to minimize interaction. But do not really go away out of his sight or out of his earshot.

What you do say should be brief, quiet, and calm. The appropriate message is usually one of your concern, your availability, and an acknowledgment of his sadness. Do not ask searching questions or try to promote a responsive conversation. An indication that the tantrum is over is often useful. Usually it is not advisable to put the child quickly back into daily events.

The "Leave-Me-Alone" stage is the end of the typical tantrum we are discussing. It may be a brief time period or may extend for several hours of relatively solitary activity by the child. Occasionally a child falls asleep during this stage. The next stage that will be discussed really concerns the aftermath of the temper tantrum proper.

Hangover

The aftermath of the tantrum varies considerably. Some children talk and look as though "nothing ever happened"—except for a little fatigue and a slight redness of the eyes or face. For lack of a better label, let us call their aftermath a "clean drunk." To all appearances, these children have "shot their wad," blown up, ventilated in the extreme, and now seem in their usual condition. Their dissociated anger outburst seems to have cleared the register for new transactions.

In contrast, other children look "hungover." Their post-upset time is marked by guilt, annoyance with self, even some self-reproach. Their complaints later may suggest efforts to externalize the guilt or project the blame for the tantrum. They complain that a favorite counselor or their therapist is always away on such-and-such a day. They imply that had their favorite (a person whose ego they can share or draw on) been around, the upset would not have occurred. They may of course be correct. A lingering post-upset depression may manifest itself as a complaint that the place is boring. These children imply that our activities did not keep them sufficiently diverted from their problems. For the hungover child, there is clearly an available memory of the tantrum and some distress over its occurrence. It may range from indirect expression of the leftover feelings to a direct self-reproach for that awful upset. When it comes to tantrums, let us be clear that we are in favor of hangovers. They make more possible the adult's efforts to teach the child some alternative to a tantrum.

Inner Dynamics and Management Suggestions. If the upset has been of the "clean-drunk" variety, it is advisable for the adult to promote a measured amount of post-tantrum awareness for the child. Much of our conversation can be directed at developing the child's awareness of the cues to the coming of the tantrum. Talking to the child about what we saw or felt that led to the tantrum helps the child to be more aware of that period of time when he missed alternative ways of dealing with his feelings.

Some mention of what the upset looked like to others can be given. It is often possible to imbed this description in comments that protect the child from the "barbs" of other children.

> The other kids were scared. You looked so wild, so miserable, so frightened. They might tease you about what happened. Do you realize how you looked? You could tell them it's over now.

Recalling other children's upsets (as part of describing tantrums in general) may create some willingness on the child's part to deal with what has happened. The goal at this point is to produce some hangover. The optimum is a mild degree of anxiety. This anxiety can be directed at a search for useful behavioral cues to the tantrum and will create a need for knowledge about alternative means of communicating distress. One hopes to be aiding in the conversion of the panic-level anxiety of the tantrum to signal anxiety that will mobilize reality-bound defenses. Of course, moving this understanding from after the tantrum to before the tantrum does not occur after one conversation. With children "addicted" to tantrums, it takes a considerable amount of time just to produce a hangover.

If you do succeed in developing a hangover (or the child had one to start with), there is other work to do. The guilt, self-image damage, and depression that constitute the hangover call for constructive help by the adult. We have referred to this help as "stitching up the tear in the ego." Reviewing the sequence of events as an attempt to call for help, a sense of hopelessness, the desperate effort to hold together, and the lonely small feeling of the calm is constructive. It helps the child see his behavior in some other light than complete "craziness" or "badness." The adult's translation of the events must *not* communicate approval but understanding. The search for a better signal of trouble-coming, the necessity of engaging an adult ally for the ego, and the learning of alternative coping skills must be emphasized. Your helpful explanations to the child should not imply that you are sure he will never have another tantrum.

The development of hangover helps to create "talkable-about-self-imagery" for the child. Adult and child begin to share communications about the tantrum. Words or phrases with a mutually understood reference develop.

That's when you went off the track. . . . That was way out. . . . That wild-man business wears you out. Do you remember all that ugly talk that led to the wildness?

The discovery of words that child and adult can agree

upon as descriptions of the lead-in behavior of the "Rumble and Grumble" are especially valuable. They may become a means of making visible to the child some feeling or piece of behavior that can function as an anxiety signal. He can come to see that "something is lost" feeling or "a black mood" as discomfort and anxiety for which he can seek help from an adult. The adult can then help the child understand and manage his feelings of ego crumble with more age-appropriate behavior than a tantrum.

A certain amount of self-image damage may result from hangover conversations. The child feels defeated because he has had one of those awful tantrums again. The helping adult should take care to focus that feeling on the "bad" act (the tantrum) and not on the "bad" person.

Summary and Implications

We have presented a set of notions to aid in the observation, understanding, and management of a typical temper tantrum. Our six stages should not be read as an invariant sequence of inevitable events. They are intended as ideas that differentiate tantrums, that guide handling of the child toward limiting or interrupting tantrums, and that increase effective communication among the adults concerned with understanding and managing the child.

Our theory represents the tantrum as a series of ego conditions. In the "Rumbling-and-Grumbling" stage, the child's ego is crumbling under the burden of growing panic. Signal anxiety is either not available at all or unable to mobilize defenses and coping skills to deal with the mounting discomfort. At the "Help-Help" stage the child externalizes the anxiety by doing something that alarms (signals) the adults around him. He does something forbidden as a signal indicating his need for help. With the arrival of adult control, the tantrumming child struggles to maintain some sense of his own ego's efficacy, or at least identity, by a series of ego retrenchments. "Either-Or" covers mainly his efforts to maintain a sense of efficacy, some sense of causing events. "No-No" is a retreat to a more primitive identity, but still maintains interpersonal contact. In the "Leave-Me-Alone" stage the retreat is from contact with others in an effort to maintain an even smaller "all-alone" me. The draining of outward aggression and the increase of depression occur mainly in these last two stages. The "Hangover" discussion focused on developing the child's awareness of what happened in the tantrum and our efforts at making alternative behavior more available to the child.

Dangers and Pitfalls

There is some danger that fascination with the various aspects of the tantrum's stages could lure one into unconsciously promoting tantrums. The "loving" attention implicit in our phenomenology could function to "reinforce" the child's tantrums. From another standpoint we might "appreciate" or "understand" tantrums so well that we come to accept them as appropriate ways of signaling for help or attention in a treatment center. Pseudo-tantrums could develop. From the child's standpoint it would be: "These people are more attentive and helpful if I put on a big upset." This is an avoidable danger. That it exists does not prove its opposite, i.e., that ignoring tantrums will make them disappear. This over-attentive situation, of course, is very different from the environment that is so callous and insensitive that only a tantrum gets adult attention.

There are, however, children who come into residential treatment after long periods in these callous environments. They may be "addicted" to tantrums as a means of affecting the environment. Even after a prolonged period of treatment, they continue to produce tantrums despite the clear availability of better ego skills. We continue to understand these tantrums carefully, limit them, even talk the child through some of them. But when stressful inner experiences or outer difficulties come about, the addicted child seems unable to keep from drinking the bottle marked "Temper Tantrum" again. With these youngsters, the danger is that we never force the issue of using some alternative to the tantrum. Our benign, skilled, treatment-oriented milieu continues to understand and manage, but finds it unpalatable to use a system of rewards and punishment to "force" the child to use his other coping skills in the stressful situation. Our experience has been that reward and punishment does work with children for whom our observation of their tantrums has been detailed and careful enough to discover the lead in behavior. Once we have that knowledge and are aware that better alternatives are available to that child, we can use rewards (praise, privileges, or natural reinforcements) for his using the better alternative and/or punishments (criticism, restriction of privileges, or absence of reinforcement) for his continuing with the tantrum (Ferster and Simons, 1966). The detailed knowledge of the child's tantrums is a prerequisite, but the consistent use of reward and punishment ("behavior modification") can speed the end of an addiction to tantrums.

Some Implications and Values

The more carefully we can observe a child's tantrum, the more likely we are able to see its individual nuances. In addition, our more complex understanding of the child in the life-space should promote variations in our management of the child. For some children we will be able to interrupt their tantrums and keep from having to push them to further ego retrenchments with our handling. For other children we may find ways of talking them through a tantrum, literally conversing about their versions of the various stages without all that flailing and wailing. The adult needs to be clear about his helpful and protective role as he does this "talking through," so this conversation is not a "one-up-I-know-all-about-you" act instead of a constructive expansion of the child's self-awareness. It takes a long standing positive relationship and a child with an "observing ego" to use "talking through" effectively.

A greater understanding of tantrums diminishes the adult's fear of them. Having various means of understanding and managing a tantrum "empowers" the adult to cope more effectively. Conversely, the tantrum or threat of tantrum loses some of its power to manipulate adults into untenable positions, and it loses some of its power to force foolish concessions from adults. The likelihood of counteraggression by the adult diminishes with alternative courses of action. In brief, understanding tantrums as a sequence of ego conditions helps to keep the adult's management within the framework of therapeutic intervention on behalf of the child. It can help us stay on the side of healthy growth and development.

A set of notions like the stages is conceptualized somewhere between the therapists' ego psychology and the child-care workers' life-space management. To the extent that it can be shared by both, it can facilitate their communication. It can aid making observations of tantrums that will be helpful to the therapists (McDermott, Fraiberg, and Harrison, 1968). In turn, it can help the child-care worker gear his management to the therapist's understanding of the child's ego. Together child-care worker and therapist can construct therapeutic interventions with the child.

We have found that the training and supervision of child-care workers is aided by life-space formulations of ego processes such as these stages of tantrums. They offer a means of going over critical incidents with the trainee. They help the worker feel that there is something organized to learn about dealing with children, even in the "uptight" situation. Skillful assessment of children before upset sensitive activities (like trips in a car) can be helped by understanding the stages of the tantrum. Of course, if tantrums in your milieu tend to occur at particular times or around particular activities, it would be wise to assess the adequacy of your routines and the fit of your program with the needs of your children.

Last of all, but most central, the child stands to gain a teacher and ally for his ego. Sensitive understanding and constructive management of the tantrum helps the child build a better ego. It may even aid him take the risks entailed in growing up—the risks of trusting others, the risks that some failures may greet his attempts at more age-appropriate coping (Bettelheim, 1967, p. 328).

Tantrums often accompany the uncertainties of a child's

new approaches to life. Unless we can help him at these times, he may give up his struggle to grow.

References

BETTELHEIM, BRUNO. 1967. *The empty fortress.* New York: Free Press.

FERSTER, C. B., and JEANNE SIMONS. 1966. Behavior: therapy with children. *Psychological Record,* 16(1): 65–71.

FREUD, SIGMUND. 1949. *An outline of psychoanalysis.* New York: W. W. Norton.

MCDERMOTT, JOHN F., SELMA FRAIBERG, and SAUL HARRISON. 1968. Residential treatment of children: the utilization of transference behavior. *Journal of the American Academy of Child Psychiatry,* 7(2): 169–192.

REDL, FRITZ, and DAVID WINEMAN. 1957. *The aggressive child.* Glencoe, Ill.: Free Press.

STONE, L. JOSEPH, and JOSEPH CHURCH. 1957. *Childhood and adolescence.* New York: Random House.

WHITE, ROBERT W. 1963. Ego and reality in psychoanalytic theory. *Psychological Issues,* Monograph II, 3(3): 1–210.

VIII
OBSERVING AND RECORDING CHILDREN'S BEHAVIOR
A Framework for the Child-Care Worker

James K. Whittaker

Why Record?

Probably no other profession has subjected its words and deeds to such a critical appraisal as has the mental health profession. For example, in the area of residential treatment for emotionally disturbed children, we not only subject our child-care workers to the rigors of an eight-hour shift with hyperaggressive, impulse-ridden children, but then expect them to write about it afterward! The essential "reason" for this compilation of detailed material is, of course, communication. In a good therapeutic residence this may mean something as mundane as "who fought with whom at recess," or something as esoteric as an analysis of some intrapsychic process. There are long- as well as short-range reasons for recording; for example, the combined efforts of many people in two or three years of residential treatment must in some way be communicated to the "significant others" in a child's life: teacher, parents, caseworkers, etc.

Basically, there are three different goals served by good

recording: *information, evaluation of progress,* and *research.* Some types of recording (e.g., diagnostic outline) are designed specifically to answer the question, "What kind of a child is this?" One of the ways the treatment plan for a child is modified is through a careful analysis of his behavior and therapeutic progress over a period of time. Thus, the skilled clinician might wish to look at a child's performance over a great many bedtimes to see if his nighttime fears have increased, decreased or remained about the same. Similarly, an analysis of the cohesiveness of the group, as well as its ability to solve problems gives us some clues as to the developmental levels of the individual children. Finally, if the long and arduous task of the child-care worker is to have any transfer value to the "outside world," daily recordings must be scrutinized in such a way that successful behavior management techniques and clinical exploitation skills are codified, written down, and passed on to other people who will be working with the child when residential treatment is terminated. One need only look to Redl and Wineman's classic, *The Aggressive Child* (1957), to see the tremendous importance of the carefully recorded and analyzed therapeutic contact.

It is the purpose of this chapter to explain in detail the four different forms of recording: *critical incident recording, individual recording, group recording,* and *behavior rating scales.* Careful attention will be paid to the question, "What should be recorded?" as well as to how the material should be organized. A final section will be devoted to exploring some pitfalls to accurate recording.

How To Organize the Material

Institutions will place different emphasis on the type of material they wish to collect and the form they will use to collect it. For example, the recording needs of a juvenile detention facility and those of a diagnostic study home for children would be quite different. The former would require, first and foremost, an up-to-date listing of the current population, as well as current medical data and any startling new or dangerous behavior exhibited by the child. The study home would require a much more thorough and detailed picture of the child which would include such information as relationships with peers, relationships with adults, response to change and management efforts, and concept of self. They would also require one ongoing report on changes in group structure and process, and they would be most interested in noting behavioral changes or critical incidents as they occurred. Finally, some institutions might be interested in simply charting the frequency and intensity of a particular behavior over a specified length of time. This behavioral rating scale would require little more than a checklist or behavioral chart. The emphasis on which form of recording to use will depend on the informational needs of the agency and the amount of time allotted for recording.

The case examples derive directly from the recording system at the Walker Home, which uses with varying emphasis all four forms of recording: individual, group, critical incident, and behavior rating scales. We present the following examples not as a recording model to be duplicated exactly by all child caring facilities, but rather as concrete illustrations of the four different forms of recording.

Critical incident recording

This data is kept in a separate notebook and contains the following kinds of information.

1. *Unsettled or unclear problems or "issues" which should be dealt with by a counselor on the incoming shift, a member of the supervising staff or the child's therapist.*

Illustration: To morning staff: Dick and Arnie had a scuffle at bedtime last night over the ownership of a fishing reel. Dick claims that he sold it to Arnie last week, but then bought it back with Arnie's approval. Arnie disputes this and says Dick merely "took it back." Staff put reel in the office and told both boys that this would be dealt with in the morning. (My hunch is that Dick's story is probably correct, but that Arnie feels somehow "gypped" or "conned" into selling the reel back. Suggest that someone get to this early, as I'm sure that Arnie and Dick will wake up, rarin' to go!)

E.B.W., 7–10–65

2. *Noteworthy incidents or interviews involving one or more children that would benefit from a more detailed process recording.*

Illustration: Re: Harold.
Evidently, last evening Harold took both sets of Caroline's keys and had hidden them behind the desk. Ostensibly, he took them because he was angry at Caroline for shutting him out of the cooking activity when he became unmanageable (fighting with Doug). Harold retrieved the keys and then proceeded to "beg" to go outside. I told him that I wanted to do some talking with him about the keys, since they were kind of a signal to him (and to us) that he was pretty worried about something. I asked specifically about home and he responded in a pretty gloomy manner: "Momma has laryngitis, Dad has headaches, is out of work," and the family was planning to move. I asked Harold what things were like at home when Dad was out of work before. "You just don't have money to buy all of the things that you want to buy, and you have to live in a place that is not so nice." He recalled a time when there had hardly been enough to eat. He would contrast this with the times before when times were good and there were skating lessons, trips to Vermont, etc. This rather idealized version of the past contained a good many fantasy elements: Harold admitted that his story about Disneyland stemmed from the fact that if he had not been sick on a particular holiday, he might have been able to go to California with his grandparents. This sounded a little like their response to his request to go to Virginia to see Nancy [1] ("if the car was O.K."). I told Harold that sometimes parents feel bad about not being able to take their kids on vacation trips and sometimes try to make their children feel that they were really the cause of their not going. . . . Back on the "key" issue, I just reiterated the events of the last few days for Harold:

> He calls home and Mom has laryngitis, can't talk and has to be interpreted by Dad. . . .
>
> Harold begins (and parents feed in) to think about the Montreal trip as if he is really going. . . .

[1] Nancy was a former counselor and a favorite of Harold's.

Miss C. (social worker) comes Monday afternoon and will more likely than not have some bad news about family (my hunch). . . .

Rosemary (counselor) "locks" Harold out of school and he breaks down part of the door to get in. . . .

Monday evening there is trouble in the kitchen and Caroline tells him he must leave. . . .

Harold takes Caroline's keys and hides them behind the desk. . . .

I said that it seemed to me that he was getting shut out of a lot of places— home, school, activities, etc.—and had this ever happened before, i.e., had he ever been "locked out" at other places. "Sometimes, when I came home, my mother would have left and she would leave a note for me telling me where the key was."

"That must have been pretty surprising, even frightening, when you came home and found that your mother was gone!"

"What I didn't like most was that she would never tell me about it and I would just come home and find her gone." I asked him if he had ever come home and found her gone with no note; he said that this had happened once and that he had gone over and stayed at his friend's house. I pointed out to him that it seemed whenever he felt that same way (being shut out), he would make sure that the adult would not (or could not) leave him by making an issue out of something, anything, so that the adult would not leave.

Comments: Two things were significant here:

1. Harold was able to relate a past feeling state (being locked out of home) with the current situation at W.H. In other words, he was acknowledging in so many words that his behavior had a purpose and was not simply random activity. He also was able to recall some of his old feelings (loneliness, confusion) and agree that this was the way he felt last night.

2. Harold was able to see (at least somewhat) that his choice of behavior was really a signal that he was getting to feel left out: the keys, the car locks, etc. I think where we go from here is to try and build in a new signal, one hopefully that is Harold's head.

J.K.W., 3–7–66

3. *Other pertinent data: notes on phone calls, home visits and life space interview summaries.*

Illustration: Larry returned from his home visit today laden with "goodies"; again, his mother had loaded him down with food of every description, as well as with two shopping bags chock full of toys. Trouble began almost as soon as Larry walked in the door: other boys wanted to see what was in the bag. I encouraged Larry to let staff put some of the food and toys away for later time. He did this, but it wasn't easy for him. Larry admitted that it would be "hard to take care of all the stuff at the same time." I used the approach that his parents had given him the things to have fun with and not to worry about. (Let's get to his social worker post-haste with a message for mother about gifts after visits!!)

J.B., 8–11–66

Often telephone calls to home provide material to talk over with the child at a later date.

Illustration: Harold called home after dinner this evening; earlier in the day he had appeared quite agitated when he learned that his family was planning to move again. His sister answered the telephone and told Harold that mother had gone to " some hotel" and that she was all alone. Later, it turned out that father was home and he did speak briefly with Harold. Bulk of conversation was spent in Harold telling sister about recent activities at W.H. Later, staff talked with Harold about problem of moving, his feeling left out of picture, etc. promised to see social worker tomorrow to set up visit. (See individual notes.)

J.B., 9–5–66

All critical incident entries are dated and initialled; space is provided in the margin for staff comment. To avoid repetition, one may refer to the individual or group recordings for a more detailed report of the incident. This type of recording is most helpful in providing day-to-day information on children. It is most often the entry that is read first when new staff are coming on duty.

4. *Additional Critical Incident Criteria*

Critical incident, of course, does not necessarily mean noisy, obviously disturbed, or disturbing behavior. A casually given new piece of *personal history* (e.g., "I remember the day my dog got killed.") can often be a critical sign of readiness to move in a new therapeutic direction. An *interesting fantasy* or softly muttered *fear* should also be considered critical incidents. One other kind of incident also has "critical" value. It is one that goes on in the adult rather than in the child's head. You might call it the *suddenly seen pattern;* e.g., "I never noticed before, but I believe Billy usually gets upset every Sunday morning or every time another boy mentions dogs, etc." Personal history, fantasies, fears, and suddenly seen patterns should all be considered critical incidents worthy of note.

Illustration: Re: Toby.

Toby woke up in a grumpy mood today and engaged in two fights with his roommates before breakfast. This has become a regular problem for him during the last week, and I talked with him after breakfast to see if I could determine the source of the difficulty. At first, he would give me no hint as to what was bothering him except to say that he had a "problem," but wasn't going to talk about it. I commented to him that he looked tired and that perhaps if he could tell me about it, he would be able to get more rest at night. At this, he shouted, "Well, you'd be tired too if that goddamn Alice [night staff] was waking you up every night." (Earlier that month, Toby had been wetting the bed and had asked staff to wake him during the night so that he would wake up dry in the morning.) "Do you mean you have a hard time getting back to sleep after this?" "Yeah, and besides it doesn't work anyway, 'cause I wet the bed again this morning." Toby then, opened up with a long conversation about what it was like to lie there awake when everybody else in the room was sleeping. It turned out that this was one of the reasons that he was having troubles in the early morning: i.e., just as he was getting to sleep, the others would be waking up and would wake Toby up in the process. This would anger him and it would usually end up in a fight. Toby also expressed a good deal of concern over a forthcoming visit home. I went over past situations where he had become worried about something and bedwetting had become more of a problem for him. I told him that I was more concerned with his getting to sleep and that for now, we would not bother about the bedwetting and let him sleep undisturbed. Toby agreed to this and felt that, for the time being, he would not mind waking up in a wet bed.

J.B., 6–17–66

Individual Recording

In individual recording we attempt to look at each child through the matrix of five major categories: the *individual child*; *relationships with peers*; *relationships with adults*; *response to change and managements*; and *handling suggestions*. The child is charted twice daily, after each shift; the emphasis is on recording relevant data and not simply writing down something to fill out each category. Again, there is no hard and fast rule about how often this type of recording should be done. Some agencies might find it sufficient to do weekly, monthly or even quarterly summaries on their children.

Our aim will be to try and illustrate the kinds of information in individual recordings, and to leave the question of "how often?" up to the individual treatment setting.

Illustration:

Date 3–6–65

Child: *Patrick*
A.M. *P.M.* X
Staff: *J.K.W.*

I. *The Individual Child*

Pat appeared quite happy when I came on duty today; he told me that today was the day he was going to buy a new baseball glove that he had been saving up for. It seems like only a few months ago when he was afraid to get in a game with the other boys. Pat spent an active afternoon and evening and fell asleep easily at 8:45.

II. *Relationships with Peers*

Pat used his new glove quite appropriately with the other boys, though he had some difficulty in not being "first" at bat. He and Gerry were vying for power in trying to decide who should be first, but Pat settled this by letting Gerry use his glove in return for letting Pat be the first one at bat. There was some mild horseplay with Danny at bedtime with Pat doing most of the initiating.

III. *Relationships with Adults*

Pat stuck pretty closely to male staff during most of the shift today with one notable exception. Shortly after lights out, he bellowed for a counselor, and when I went into his room, he said that only Mary would do. Mary went in shortly and Pat showed her a fairly large blister that had developed on the sole of his foot. It is not unusual for Pat to seek out female staff when he has some somatic complaint, particularly when they occur around bedtime. I've noticed that Pat is joining more and more into activities with the other boys, he is spending less time seeking out one to one relationships with staff.

IV. *Response to Change and Management Efforts*

I had to limit Pat tonight at bedtime when he began to try to make loud noises during the story. He tried for a while to get Danny involved in this when it was fairly obvious that Danny was trying to get to sleep. I found that direct appeal served to quiet him down, saying both that Danny was tired and wanted to go to sleep and that his making noises made it very difficult for the other boys to listen to the story.

V. *Handling Suggestions*

I think it would be wise to think of some parallel activities for Pat and Gerry, since neither one of them seems to be able to handle direct and open competition. Perhaps staff can suggest to Pat some other activities besides baseball (perhaps woodworking?). I think the novelty of this game will begin to wear thin after a while, particularly if he is competing with Gerry who is so much better than he is.

Obviously, if individual recording is done over longer periods of time, it will include a more detailed picture of the child's growth and changes in his development. At Walker Home, individual cases are usually summarized twice yearly using the daily recordings as the primary data.

Group Recording

Typically, group recordings consist of a very brief tonal picture of a group for a given shift. Each group recording contains at least the following information: major group activities, significant group events (runaways, group projects, etc.), changes in group structure (power structure, leadership structure, activity structure), and significant group processes (ranking, scapegoating). These daily group recordings are supplemented periodically by a more detailed analysis of group structure and processes. This latter type of recording might be done simply with the idea of getting a picture of the group over periods of time, or it might be carried out with a specific problem focus: e.g., an analysis of the realignment of the power structure after a new boy's arrival. The basic purpose of the daily group recordings is to provide us with a concise picture of what the group is like for a particular time period. Counselors read the daily group notes almost like a barometer, before they go on duty.

Example: Total group engaged in some cohesive activity around skating, but when the others were ready to leave, Tim refused to get off the ice. Mike, Al, and Pete began calling names at him and threatening him with harm if he didn't hurry up. Back at Walker, boys were rather lethargically watching television and Tim sank into the television oblivion which took the heat off him somewhat. Before lunch today, little subgroups were going especially strong. Jeff and H's subgroup deteriorated when H. lost interest in J.'s new cabinet. Children seem to be drifting from group to group without too much thought as to the pertinence of the subgroup. There were no major group upsets, though there may well be if Tim continues to set himself up against the total group.

R.A.S., 1–14–67 P.M.

Behavior Rating Scale

This last form of recording is used to indicate the presence or absence of a particular behavior. It is the most predetermined form, in the sense that what is sought is specified before it actually happens. Simple behavior rating scales may be completed simply by checking off the appropriate category. For example:

1.	Frequently seen	Seldom seen	Absent
Nail biting	X		
Eye tic		X	
Facial grimace		X	
Hand wringing			X
Eye rolling			X
Head banging			X

2.	Fighting	Fire setting	Destroying property
Joe	X		
Tim	X		
Arny	X		
Howard		X	X
Alan	X		
Sam	X		

Other scales may seek to obtain data on a particularly problematic situation; for example, the following scale was used to learn more about the counselor's response to a particularly troublesome behavior, and the child's reaction to the management technique.

Illustration:

(A) *Presenting behavior:* Joe told Sam to go fuck himself this morning, as soon as he came in for breakfast.

(B) *Counselor response:* I told Joe to cut it out, or he would have to leave the room.

(C) *Child's reaction:* Joe laughed and said he was only "fooling"; I told him that nobody liked to be greeted that way.

Using a simple scale like the above one, it is possible to factor analyze the various management techniques pertaining to a particular "issue" and the degree of success they achieved.

One of the obvious problems in working with a checklist system is to define the categories in such a way that the observers are all agreed upon what constitutes the specific behavior to be charted. For example, if recording the frequency of a "temper tantrum," the observer had better be quite clear as to exactly what behavior constitutes a "temper tantrum." The greater the number of observers, the greater the problem becomes.

What To Record

The whole question of what to record is often one that throws the new worker into a state of mild panic. "How can I ever remember everything that happened?" is usually the first question asked by the novice child-care worker. The answer, of course, is that no one can "remember" everything that happened, and, indeed, to attempt to write such a complete daily chart on each child would make a cumbersome report to read. Finally, good observing and recording skills must develop over time; the process of developing insight into what is clinically significant behavior must develop in the same way as the clinical management skills of the counselor. This section will raise a series of questions to be asked about individual children and groups of children. The answers to these questions are expected to give substance to the outlines of the four different forms of recording presented in the second section. Clearly, how many questions are to be answered will be determined in a large part by the scope of the recording task; thus, a six-months' report will contain a far more detailed analysis than an individual daily recording. Special attention will be given to individual and group recording, as both of these have direct relevance for critical incident recording.

The following material is based on the recording outline developed by David Wineman for the University of Michigan Fresh Air Camp. This outline has been supplemented in certain sections, by some of the questions found to be useful by the Walker Home staff.

Redl has devised another recording outline (1966, pp. 333–337) consisting of ten headings under which a child-care worker can organize his thoughts about the individual child. In neither case are the outlines meant to be used as a rigid model to be followed scrupulously for each child; rather, they are intended to be used as helpful guidelines to give the task of recording some direction.

Individual Recording Form

I. *The Individual Child*

a. Physical description of the child including general appearance, grooming, manner of dress and habits of cleanliness.
b. "Atmospheric" elements, such as facial expressions, mood-peculiar mannerisms, gait, manner of speech, intelligence, etc.
c. How does he seem to view himself? Does he think he is

lucky? Unlucky? Does he see himself as good? Bad? Is he fatalistic in regard to his behavior? His future?

d. What does his value system appear to be? Is he identified with "middle class" values, delinquent values or others? How are these value positions expressed? How deeply imbedded are his values? Are there conflicts between them? Does he show guilt? At what times and in what way?

e. What is his ability to tolerate frustration? What types of frustration are more difficult or less difficult for him? How does he react to frustration?

f. Indicate insights into his fantasy life, day dreams, future goals, and ambitions. What kinds of stories and comics is he attracted to? What fantasy roles does he like to play?

g. Does he have any particular fears? Unusually strong interest in some particular activity or stereotyped avoidance? Are there any striking habits that appear peculiar or out of the ordinary?

h. How much control does he seem to have over his behavior? Do controls break down under certain conditions? What are they?

i. What kind of a self image does he have? What does he think his assets and liabilities are? What does he see as his biggest problem? What does he think is the best thing about him? The worst?

j. How does he deal with hurt, anger, sadness, and joy?

k. What is the character of his anger? For example, is it chronic annoyance, or emotional flare-ups?

l. What have been the changes between the beginning of treatment and now?

II. *Response to Activities*

a. What is his general response to activities—enthusiastic, bored, excited etc.?

b. What activities is he attracted to: those entailing infantile gratifications, adult-like activities, activities with high fantasy content, dangerous activities? Which does he avoid? Is there a preference for activities that are more individual or that require considerable interaction with peers?

c. What is his general skill level? Is he especially adept at any particular craft or activity?

d. Are there activities he characteristically turns to when he is sad or lonely?

III. *Relationships with Peers*

a. What kinds of responses does he seek from peers? What does he do to get them? How successful is he and how does he react when he obtains the response he seeks? How does he react when that response is denied? Does he seek power? Affection? Submission?
b. What types of children does he seem closer to? Which does he avoid? How friendly is he with other children? How is the friendliness expressed? What types of children does he come into conflict with and how is the conflict expressed?
c. What seems to be his perception of other children? Is he accurate in judging the motives of other children? When is he inaccurate?
d. Does he seem to need other children? Is he content to be alone? How often and under what conditions?
e. How do the other children react to him? View him? Is he popular? Respected? Feared? Ignored? Is there a general consensus among the children in their attitudes toward him?
f. Does he seem to show any sexual interest in his peers? How strongly is this interest shown and how frequently?
g. Is he attracted to any particular subgroups? What are their characteristics?
h. What are his skills in approaching other children? In avoiding them? In influencing them? In being influenced by them?
i. Does he have difficulties functioning in large groups? What kinds of difficulties?
j. What changes have you seen between the beginning of treatment and now?

IV. *Relationship to Adults*

a. Much of what was outlined under "relationship with peers" applies here as well.
b. How comfortable is he in seeking help, encouragement, affection from adults? What form does it take? Does he have favorites among counselors? What seems to be the basis of his choice? (Male, Female, Older, Younger, etc.).
c. Is he generally obedient or defiant? What is the quality of his obedience or defiance? How does he show it? Are there differences in whom he will listen to? How does he express aggression and how frequently is he aggressive? Are there certain times or conditions during which he becomes more aggressive or defiant? How does he behave afterwards? Sulky? Worried? Hostile? Friendly?

d. How does he seem to make you and the other counselors feel toward him? How does he try to make you act? Does he succeed?
e. How accurate is his perception of adult motives and actions toward him. Under what conditions are the perceptions more or less accurate?
f. Has he expressed any sexual interest toward the counselors? Toward the males? Females? How strong does this interest appear and what form does it usually take?
g. What is his characteristic manner of showing affection for adults? Hostility?
h. What changes have you seen between the beginning of treatment and now?

V. *Response to Change and Management Efforts*

a. What management techniques seem to work best to get him to comply? Which ones seem to reduce defiance in the life space situation?
b. What seems to be the effect of insight-oriented discussions? Does he appear interested in cultivating insight into his problems?
c. What is his reaction to power squeezes and threats?
d. Does the use of program activities or peer group pressures appear to be influential in limiting his behavior? We refer here to the short term management of his behavior.
e. What is his reaction to limits? Does it make a difference who is setting them? Does it make a difference whether or not they are being applied to the group, or to him alone?
f. In general, how does he handle the structure of the day: the rules, the routines, the activities? Are there particular rules, routines, or activities which give him special difficulty (e.g., bedtime, mealtime, etc.)?

These categories were originally designed to form the basis for a final report that would accompany a child at the end of a therapeutic camping session. In a therapeutic residence, it could easily be used to constitute a quarterly or six-months' report. The child-care worker may keep the outline in mind while he is doing his daily individual recording. Beyond this, the "slant" of the daily reports will very much reflect the current behavior of the child; thus, if Joe is having all sorts of difficulties with female staff, the emphasis of the report will be heavily centered around the questions having to do with "Relationships with Adults."

The more specific the counselor can become in his recording, the more benefit it will have for the reader; for example the statement that "Joe reacted very negatively today to limit setting and engaged in several aggressive outbursts" leaves the reader with many unanswered questions: What kind of limits were being set? How were they presented? By whom? What was Joe's position in the group at the time? What does "aggressive outburst" mean?

One final note about individual recording: a good record should raise as many questions as it answers. The child-care worker should not feel responsible for giving the "definitive" answer to any of the questions in the preceding outline. Indeed, if the records are used properly the critical interchange between child-care staff often produces the most fruitful insights into the child's pathology.

Group Recording

Most group-recording outlines were designed either for the evaluation of a group over long periods of time or for the detailed analysis of a single group meeting (usually conducted by a professional social group worker).[2] While there certainly exists a need for both kinds of information in a therapeutic residence, neither model seems to fit the daily group recording needs of the child-care worker. In our earlier discussion, we defined group recording as "a brief tonal picture" of the group for a particular shift. It is intended to give a concise and accurate view of the mood and structure of the group; it is typically read like a "barometric report" by the incoming counselor. When read over a period of time, these daily reports should give us an idea of major shifts in group structure, degree of "groupness," and ability to solve problems. The fol-

[2] A notable exception to these two types of group recording forms is the one developed by Fritz Redl in *When We Deal with Children* (1966, pp. 338–345). Redl's outline is free from cumbersome jargon and is very much geared to the daily needs of the child care staff.

lowing model has been found to be useful in organizing daily group records:

I. *Major Group Activities*

The chief function of this category is simply to reduce the chances of "loading" the system with too many of the same kinds of activities. It will also tell us something of the group's ability to handle certain kinds of activities.

II. *Group Structure*

The first question to be answered here is "*Who* did *what* with *whom*?" This is often the first place where we begin to notice the formation of certain subgroups within the larger cottage culture. Certain "structures" will be watched more closely at different times in the life of the group; for example, a discharge of two high-status members would mean an almost certain realignment of the power structure. Some other questions to be answered under this heading are: "What is the group's ability to handle issues and problems?" "What kinds of controls are the children to exercise on each other?" "What particular affectional bonds seem to be developing between pairs or subgroups of children?" "Who are the group's current leaders? Scapegoats? Low status members?"

III. *Group Processes*

In what manner is the group dealing with disappointments and changes in the routine? What is nature and frequency of "ranking," cursing, and scapegoating? To whom is this behavior usually directed?

IV. *Mood of the Group*

What has the group been like to work with today? Have they been overly demanding, industrious, defiant, bothersome, "groupy," separated, provocative, or lethargic? An accurate picture of the "group atmosphere" can save the incoming child care staff immense amounts of time and trouble if they can plan for it in advance.

Some Pitfalls to Good Recording

As in any form of recording, there is always some discrepancy between the event as it actually happened and the manner in which it is transcribed. The following suggestions are offered in the hope that they might help to improve the accuracy of the recording without lessening its diagnostic implications, or limiting its style. I am indebted to Dr. Marvin Silverman whose thoughts about recording formed the basis for many of the following suggestions. Some of these may be looked upon as "pitfalls" to be studiously avoided, others as helpful hints to be incorporated into one's observing and recording skills.

1. Turning the daily log into a "gripe sheet" is an easy trap to fall into; individual supervisory conferences and staff meetings are perhaps more appropriate contexts for airing our grievances with each other and with the children. One is reminded of Erving Goffman's description of the "paper shadow" which follows the mental patient throughout his entire institutional life. We should, of course, exercise discretion in putting down our feelings about a child; this kind of information is valuable, but remember that you have a responsibility to state the child's "case" as well as your own.

Example: Tim had a totally bad morning; he was into trouble all over the place and just wasn't quiet for a minute. He was just obnoxious and kept asking for things in that real whiny way of his.

2. Overgeneralizing or being overly specific is another trap that the child-care worker might fall into. For example, nobody "constantly" fights or "always" gets into trouble. Similarly, the observer can dwell too long on the minutiae in the situation and miss the forest for the trees.

3. A merely chronological account of what a child did for an entire day simply does not tell us very much. It might be better to pick the most salient, or critical, feature in a child's day and record on that alone, rather than to outline *what* he did just to follow the outline.

4. If you use psychoanalytic terminology, be sure you know what the words mean. "Anxiety," "defense," and "acting out" are words with specific meanings. Also, be careful about

words like "infantile," "immature," and "delinquent," which may mean different things to different people. As a general rule, it is better to avoid cumbersome phraseology and the use of clinical language and simply state what the child did or said; for example, instead of "made a demonstration of positive feeling toward the counselor," you could say, "he put his arm around the counselor."

5. Each setting has a jargon of its own that is often difficult for the outsider to understand.

Example: Today, Wiley got *bumped* [asked to leave] from *O.T.* [occupational therapy] and was sent upstairs to the *Q.R.* [quiet room], where waited for the *C.S.* [charge staff]. Staff had a long *LSI* [life-space interview] with him and *rubbed him hard* [spoke firmly about a specific behavior] about *Playing the Dozens* [calling another boy's family into disrepute] with Sammy during the morning.

6. Exotic punctuation should also be avoided.

Example: Albert really made some gains today in school!!!!!!! His what-the-hell-do-I-care-anyway attitude was just not present???

7. Be careful about the use of the word "able." It carries the implication that a person now has the ability to do something that he formerly could not do. It is correct to say that a former shallow-water swimmer was able to pass his deep water test; but to say that a child was "able" to form a relationship implies that this was previously impossible for him to do.

8. Use behavioral illustrations carefully. They are most appropriate when a more general statement somehow fails to capture the essence of what you are trying to say.

Example: Billy almost seemed to be setting himself up as the scapegoat tonight; during dinner he began to dribble food on the table and make vulgar noises until finally Tommy and Winslow began to kick him under the table and had to be physically restrained from attacking him.

9. The recording of clinical "hunches," or hypotheses, or

offering behavioral interpretations is a valuable adjunct to process recording. These remarks should be set off from the process material in such a way that reader is able to easily discern what is factual and what is conjecture.

Example: Toby woke up quite angry this morning and got into a fight with Tim before breakfast. (I think this might have had something to do with the fact that Toby had wet the bed the night before and was feeling pretty upset about it.)

10. Counselors should be careful to divide recording responsibilities in such a way that they are not always charting on the same child. This will tend to serve the children better and provide more breadth of experience to the staff.

11. Recording is a developed skill that takes time to perfect and master. It is not necessary that the counselor "remember" everything that happened, as he will spend more time "remembering" than he will serving the children. Also, it is good to develop a sense of selectivity about what one records, as all behavior does not carry the same significance. Practically speaking, it is not a good idea to take notes while on duty as this will often lead to trouble and is very difficult for the children to understand. The children will all know that some kind of records are kept and the most simple and honest answer to their questions seems to be, "We keep records so that we may help all children better by being able to understand them." We must stress the confidential nature of the records with children and make it clear that they are not "bad lists" to be shared with parents, or family.

12. Unless you are making a direct quotation, avoid use of slang, i.e., "kids," or "the child 'took off.' "

13. Particularly with records that might leave the agency, we should be careful about assuming that the relationship *we* had with a child was representative of the relationships he had with *all* the adults in the setting.

14. There is nothing wrong about being puzzled about the meaning of a child's behavior. You are not expected to know everything.

Example: Carl burst into tears tonight after supper and was comforted by staff; he couldn't give any reasons for the behavior except to say that "the kids are buggin' me." Can someone shed some light on this?

15. Give consideration to the space that you allot to each point in recording. A whole page of discussion will by volume alone make a particular point seem central to the report. Watch the length of your report: Long rambling reports are not read as carefully as short concise ones.

16. Above all, respect the confidential nature of any report. This is not casual material to be discussed with friends or anyone else who is not directly connected with the child. The ultimate success, or failure, of the child's total treatment is in large measure dependent upon the quality of the reports that accompany him along the way.

References

REDL, FRITZ. 1966. Just what am I supposed to observe. In *When we deal with children.* New York: Free Press.

———, and DAVID WINEMAN. 1957. *The aggressive child.* Glencoe, Ill.: Free Press.

IX
AVOIDING SOME OF THE ROADBLOCKS TO THERAPEUTIC MANAGEMENT

Larry K Brendtro

We have long been aware that certain children require the type of total care, management, and treatment that can only be provided in a residential institution. Yet, only recently have we begun to do something about the great gulf that exists between institutionalizing a child and establishing a truly therapeutic treatment program for him. While most of the formerly custodial institutions have become at least nominally "treatment oriented" through the addition of a few mental health professionals, there has usually been very little change in the procedures that are carried out by "on-line" staff in the living situation. Child-care workers have often been provided with only minimal training and have received sporadic supervision by professionally trained personnel who experience difficulty in communicating their theories to workers in the action setting (Carducci, 1962). In the final analysis, child-care workers have generally been sent out into the milieu with little more than their own intuitive knowledge; it is little wonder that their well-meant efforts have sometimes fallen short of providing for the many and complex needs of maladjusted youth.

Numerous pressures influence the interactions between

child-care workers and the children with whom they work. Some of these pressures emanate from the cottage subculture (Mayer, 1958; Polsky, 1962) or from the organizational structure of the institution; others are the result of the personality of the worker or of those with whom he must deal. Even the most conscientious worker finds it difficult at times to cope with these pressures without interfering with the therapeutic treatment of children. The best interests of the children are sometimes forgotten as the worker strives to satisfy his own superiors, his co-workers, or the institutional policy. Even such seemingly innocent concerns as striving to control children, gaining their acceptance, and achieving success are not without their pitfalls. In this chapter we shall consider seven major issues that should be carefully considered by the child-care worker who is committed to maintaining "the therapeutic stance."

Those professionals oriented primarily toward individual psychotherapy will perhaps interpret these issues as examples of subtle or obvious "counter-transference phenomena." However, it would be a mistake to consider them only in the light of individual personality dynamics. To say of a worker that he should "get some therapy" or that "his counter-phobic stance toward danger makes children unsafe" functions mainly as a rationale for avoiding an honest look at the pressures and pitfalls of child-care work. In our experience seven issues are encountered in most institutions by most child-care workers. Often we have found that being made aware of the issues themselves enables the worker to function more effectively. Awareness and discussion of these pressures and pitfalls in child-care work is surely more helpful to most individuals than instant diagnosis and on-the-spot interpretation therapy.

The Need to Conform to Institutional Policy [1]

It might seem that the most important determinant of the in-

[1] For sake of discussion we shall refer to the pressures confronting the child-care personnel as "needs" of the worker. This is a general usage of the term and should not necessarily imply the meaning associated with the more formal motivation construct of the "needs."

teraction between a child-care worker and the children for whom he is responsible would be the formal policy of the institution. This would include the numerous written and unwritten expectations that delineate the role of the child-care worker in that particular institution and govern his relationships with the children and with other staff members. For example, most institutions restrict the child-care staff from using corporal punishment as a means of discipline; on a more general level the institution may expect that the child-care workers "accept" all of the children in their charge, without spelling out how this is done or even what it means. Because of the gulf between the formal policies of many institutions and the daily experience of the child-care staff, these formal policies may exert relatively little influence on the actual staff-child interaction. As Grossbard (1960) suggests, the directives of the administration often stop at the cottage door.

The depth of influence of institutional policy varies with the amount of supervision and the rigidity with which the policy is supported by sanction (e.g., does a worker ever lose his job for hitting a child?). But, regardless of the formal policy, there is in practice always a great deal of leeway available to the child-care worker. It is relatively easy to maintain a superficial compliance to gross institutional policy ("don't buck the system") without necessarily modifying one's ideas and practices to correspond to the expectations of superiors. If confrontation ever does become imminent, the worker still has a variety of alternatives: (1) agreeing with and following the supervisor's suggestion for change; (2) publicly agreeing but later ignoring the suggestion of the supervisor; (3) pointing out that what is suggested has actually been done all along: "why, we have been doing that for years"; and (4) pointing out that the suggestion is welcome but not practical: "that won't work because . . ." or "we tried that once but. . . ."

The foregoing is not to suggest that child-care workers thrive on deceptive noncompliance with the expectations of superiors and are patently dishonest, or are consciously building an "underground" organization, attempting to undermine the policies of the institution. Rather, these observations are in accord with the suggestion that although lofty proclamations of institutional policy certainly have some effect, their influence is considerably less than is commonly thought. In order to preserve his position, the child-care worker must, of necessity, overtly comply with at least some of the prescribed institutional policies; beyond this he is often on his own, with his performance determined by his own ideas, needs, and other pressures upon him.

It is also possible for the worker to "hide behind" the policy of the institution or his distorted interpretation of such a policy. Thus, the disinterested child-care worker may coldly apply rigid institutional standards to the children's behavior because "these are the rules," while a fearful or insecure worker often responds with "well, I don't mind myself, but you know what the policy is." At the other end of the continuum, a passive, lazy, or irresponsible worker may all too willingly conform to an institutional policy of "permissiveness." Likewise, the worker who becomes excessively anxious when forced to confront aggressive youngsters with their behavior may grasp some institutional policy that supposedly justifies his "acceptance" of such behavior.

The Need to Satisfy Supervisors and Superiors

The child-care worker functions within an institutional power structure where administrative and clinical personnel usually have most of the authority (Mayer, 1963).

Whether the child-care worker is subordinate to numerous others in the institution or has some measure of autonomy, he quickly learns which people within the organization are powerful and, more specifically, which ones hold his job "in their hands." He may, by means of the always existent institutional grapevine, become aware of former workers who have had to leave because of difficulties around particular issues or with particular authority figures. The worker soon realizes that his welfare (pay increases, time off, subtle privileges) will be fostered only if he pleases these authority figures.

More so than any other employee of the institution, the child-care worker is vulnerable to the "fishbowl" phenomena.

Although nobody would dare to wander into the sanctity of the therapy hour, many child-care workers feel they must be constantly "on guard" lest some superior wander in at an inopportune moment and "gets the wrong idea." Only the most confident worker is insensitive to the presence of administrative or clinical personnel in his cottage or area of the institution. There may even develop a system of communication wherein workers "warn" one another of approaching authority. This warning is generally followed by a scurry of activity and "appropriate behavior" that is demonstrable evidence of the worker's need to impress his superiors.

In one institution, the director had a definite opinion about staff competition with children in competitive sports, such as basketball or football. The gratification staff derived from such interaction was too great to be suppressed by the director's beliefs, and the workers participated vigorously in such games. But whenever the director's automobile was seen approaching the playing field, someone would shout "time to referee" and all staff players suddenly became referees until it was again safe to rejoin the activity.

One particularly significant problem that can result from the need to please supervisors centers around the control of acting-out behavior. Supervisors may convey the impression (or fact) that job effectiveness is inversely related to the number of discipline problems that come to light. The cottage with marred doors, broken furniture, or fighting boys is often seen as incriminating an ineffective worker. The fact that some of such behavior is to be expected when working with aggressive, maladjusted youngsters (or with "normal" children, as any parent might attest) does not need elaboration. Nevertheless, this behavior causes the worker to become anxious lest his effectiveness be questioned. He often overreacts to the negative behavior, thus missing the opportunity to deal therapeutically with this problem. In his attempt to suppress misbehavior, the worker may become extremely "jumpy" about minor issues.

A child-care worker approached an adolescent who was a chronic behavior problem. The youngster was watching television quietly, with his feet propped up on a chair. The worker jerked out the chair, saying that he "needed" it. The boy looked irritated, but quietly found another older wooden chair for his "footstool." The worker again came over, jerked out the chair, and grumbled something about "what Dr. S. would think if he came in and saw the kids with their feet all over the furniture."

This is a minor incident and is perhaps not in and of itself extremely deleterious to the development of the youngster; however, when multiplied by numerous such incidents it may foster an environment considerably less than therapeutic.

The Need To Be Accepted by Co-Workers

In all except the smallest of institutions there are several people of a "peer" level with whom a worker must interact. There develops a type of subculture among these individuals who share common problems, tasks, and frustrations. We have become aware of the importance of the "subculture of the gang" as it applies to our work with delinquents. However, we may have overlooked the influence of the "subculture of the child-care workers" within our institution.

In the ideal situation, the norms and values held by the workers are highly compatible with the goals of the institution and the total treatment philosophy. The notions about the treatment milieu, theories of child management, and the role of the various professionals and non-professionals in the institution are generally accepted by all concerned. Such broad consensus on means and ends contributes to a smoothly running treatment organization. In practice, unfortunately, this situation seldom exists. For example, the overall formal policy on corporal punishment might clearly prohibit this means of disciplinary control; the child-care staff, on the other hand, may feel that at times it is necessary to "knock them back in line" or to "show them who is running the show." This is not meant to imply that brutality is rampant in all or most children's institutions. Rather, certain underlying values, attitudes, and practices develop among the child-care staff which are at odds with the formal policies of the institution. Thus, it is important to the worker that he be perceived by his colleagues as competent in his job. Since child behavior is usually thought to be the prime indicator of worker inadequacy, the competent worker is the one who exercises high control over his charges, is quite authoritarian, and suppresses any acting-out behavior. It is not uncommon to see workers to go to great lengths to demonstrate their "behavior control prowess" to one another, often to the detriment of the children.

Two child-care workers were outside a dormitory room after "lights out," and several of the boys inside were laughing, joking, and making considerable noise. One worker said to the other, "Watch how they shape up when I come on the scene!" He then burst through the doorway, flicking on the lights, and shouted, "I can't even walk down the hall a minute without you nuts acting like a bunch of idiots!" Then, singling out two likely culprits, he continued shouting "Get down to the dayroom and sit until you can act decent!" One complied guiltily, but the other boy screamed back, "Don't shout at me!" and proclaimed his innocence. After a few sharp verbal interchanges with the child-care worker, the boy obliged, running down to the dayroom, sobbing, "I was just an innocent bystander . . . just an innocent bystander."

Regardless of the formal orientation the institution provides for new workers, the "old guard" soon conveys many of its own attitudes through a more informal yet highly effective "orientation." This may include anything from casual remarks to the planful disappearance of the regular staff at a moment of great crisis so that "the new guy can see what these kids are really like."

An older child-care worker was heard "joking" with a new, more flexible, and highly motivated worker. "Think you are going to establish *relationships* with *them*? That relationship stuff is OK as far as it goes; but what are you going to do when one of them kicks you in the teeth and says 'up yours,' huh?"

It is easy to see how the new worker, still unsure of what is expected of him and desiring to get along with his co-workers is extremely vulnerable to being enveloped by the traditional sub-rosa attitudes and practices of the established child-care worker subculture.

The Need To Adhere to Personal Philosophy

The worker's approach to children may be influenced by his philosophical or religious outlook, or by his "objective" intellectual ideas about human behavior. Each of these can in turn be determined by other aspects of an individual's personality. Thus, a particular religious orientation can be the motive that brings a person into the helping field, but, if too narrow or rigid, it can prevent the worker from being objective and flexible in the handling of deviant behavior. Some child-care workers find it very difficult to handle the threat impulsive behavior presents to their own philosophy of life and value system. They are apt to be in danger of rejecting the disturbed child as well as his disturbing behavior.

An individual committed to a philosophy of "permissiveness" or of "structure" in his approach to children may blindly hold to one narrow method and therefore be incapable of meeting the challenge presented by the complex behavior and needs of maladjusted youth. It is imperative that all who work with disturbed children make an honest attempt to assess the degree to which their own philosophical outlook is determined by their unique personality rather than the needs of disturbed children. It has been suggested that persons with inordinately strong needs for affiliation tend to develop theories that place great emphasis upon the therapeutic value of establishing a "dependency relationship," while others who fear close ties develop theories that espouse the value of avoiding "over-involvement" and fostering independence in children.

Some mention should be made of the worker who is more sophisticated in his intellectual understanding of human behavior. As our awareness of the significance of the role of the child-care worker has increased, more of these individuals have found their way into the child-care worker role, often in preparation for an eventual career in social work, psychology, or special education. Although such bright, young people can be a tremendous asset to any treatment program, their presence is not without problems. Their overintellectualized approach to working with children has been known to result in nonspontaneity of adult behavior that hampered interaction between worker and child. On numerous occasions the author has observed such an individual standing immobilized, analyzing the "sociometric patterns" or the "sympton expression" as a group of children were wildly engaged in the near destruction of one another, when the appropriate action would have been immediate intervention of any kind. A worker with some background in "psychology" is apt to feel the need to "diagnose" the children with whom he works. While the worker may be aware of the characteristic symptoms, prognosis, etc., of the various categories of mental illness, his handling of this child may be disturbed by his superficial understanding of the complex issues involved.

The child-care workers had pretty much agreed that Tim was a "sociopath" and they had read that treatment was not effective with such patients. They gave up trying to work closely with him because they all "know" sociopaths "couldn't form relationships." The best way to handle such a person was to never let him get out of line. Nobody cared to spend any time with him, and they were all speculating about how long it would be until he was "shipped out." Within a few weeks (after an attempted suicide and runaway attempt, both of which were sequels to the punitive use of isolation), Tim was transferred to the state hospital. Rather than entertain the possibility that the workers' approach had somehow contributed to Tim's problems, they reassured themselves that they "had been right all along."

The Need to Control

Control and management of disturbed children is a large and important part of the duties of child-care workers, and there are few who would currently defend the worker who was unable or unwilling to exercise appropriate controls over disturbed children. Yet, in much the same manner as a former alcoholic may become an activist in temperance work to regulate his own drinking behavior, so too a child-care worker may hold his own antisocial impulses in check by exercising control over impulsive children. This reaction formation may be of such severity as to hamper seriously the attainment of therapeutic goals. Whenever the child does the "least little thing" he finds an angry adult "jumping all over him." Depending upon the degree to which the child externalizes or internalizes these conflicts, he may develop perceptions of all adults as punitive and rejecting or of himself as unworthy and hopeless.

Bromberg (1961) has suggested that our own unconscious aggressive and rebellious impulses are projected onto those individuals who, because of their antisocial behavior, have already been marked by society. Hence, the emotional callousness and antisociability of deviant individuals is fashioned, to some extent at least, by the public's attitude toward them. We may, at the same time vicariously take pleasure in the child's negative behavior, yet we consciously ask him to reform. The worker who is identified with the acting-out behavior of the child communicates, through the use of subtle verbal and nonverbal cues, that negative behavior is expected. Whether the child is actually aware of our ambivalence, he usually gets the message and lives up to the expectations; both his negative behavior and his social distance from adults are maintained. Further documentation of the two faces of this "need to control" is seen in the almost delinquent excitement evidenced by certain workers as they relate the wild escapades of their charges. The same behavior that is righteously controlled in the cottage later becomes the source of fascinating tales related to others inside and outside of the institution. Language that would otherwise never be used by these socially respectable adults is suddenly legitimized, since they are only relating "what the children said."

It is sometimes a moot question whether the child-care workers change the behavior of disturbed children more than the children change the behavior of the child-care workers.

The Need for Success with a Child

All child-care workers need to experience a certain degree of success in their work with disturbed children; this is in addition to the need for approval by supervisors and colleagues. For the maintenance and enhancement of self-esteem, the worker must believe that he possesses some ability to work with and to help children. As with the other previously discussed needs, this concern is not detrimental in and of itself, but can be so if it exerts a disproportionate influence on worker behavior.

Certain individuals with rather pronounced personal inadequacies seek employment working with disturbed children, apparently so that by helping others with their problems, they may help themselves. Such a person is apt to place excessive emphasis on success. He is hypersensitive about whether there is any "movement" or progress in the children to whom he is assigned, and his own self-esteem may be threatened by the child with whom success does not readily come.

The person with strong needs for visible, rapid success is apt to experience considerable difficulty in long-term interaction with persistently misbehaving, adult-defiant youth. This individual may exert a vigorous effort to "help" such a child but increasingly experiences the lack of improvement as a personal threat. For a time, he may redouble his efforts to "get through" to this youngster; all of this attention may be very overwhelming to the youth, who may entrench himself further behind his adult-avoidance defenses. More than likely, the worker will soon turn his attention away from (reject) this youngster and focus upon those with whom success is more readily attainable.

Another variation along these lines is the person who persists until he finally establishes a beginning relationship with the difficult child. Once having achieved this, he turns his attention to more challenging and personally gratifying frontiers rather than becoming involved in the slow and often painful process of advancing from the relationship beachhead in pursuit of long-term treatment goals.

It would seem that the magnitude of the job of rehabilitating maladjusted children would serve to eliminate personal jealousies and feuding. Quite in contrast, all too often different workers are found vigorously competing among themselves for the individual children, each striving for success (or affection) in their work with the child. While such competition may be in accord with the general goals of a free enterprise society, it can be seriously detrimental to the needs of a child in residential treatment.

The Need to be Accepted by the Children

For many child-care workers, this touches upon one of the most central concerns in their interaction with children: the need to be accepted and liked by the children is perhaps the strongest motive that operates to bring people into this field and keep them on the job. Lest what follows be misinterpreted, we repeat again that there is "nothing wrong" with this motive in and of itself, unless it comes to override the needs of individual children. In such a situation it frequently interferes with therapeutic handling and contaminates the worker-child interaction. In its most exaggerated form it has been referred to by Horney (1937) and Reik (1963) as a neurotic need for love.

Problems around the excessive need to be accepted by children are most evident among new child-care workers who are working with children for the first time. It is also seen commonly in workers who have few outside ties, interests, or interpersonal relationships. To one degree or another this concern is shared by almost all workers.

The child-care worker's need for acceptance by the child may cause him to push a child too quickly and too deeply into a very strong relationship, implying that this relationship supersedes any attachments the child might happen to have elsewhere. Many new workers ignore the warnings of more experienced child-care personnel who caution them to "beware of over-involvement." Such a worker is apt to disregard these suggestions by others as resulting from a "lack of interest" in the children. He then sets out to "rescue" the child by the relationship he offers, only to discover some time later that he has promised the child more than he can or should deliver.

The worker may experience a child's reluctance to change and the persistence of misbehavior as a personal rebuff: "That boy dared to do that to me after all that I have done for him.

What gratitude!" The adult whose own needs are so readily frustrated soon loses his therapeutic stance.

Child-care workers may react to the aloofness of the relationship-wary youngster in varying manners. He may intensify his "wooing" to such a degree that the youth feels certain that his defenses are necessary for self-preservation. Or he may overtly or subtly reject the child, proving to the youth that he was really right all along in warding off the adult rather than trusting him. Finally, the worker may react to the "bottomless pit" of constantly giving attention to a child and receiving little or nothing in return; he simply gets tired of investing energy in the child without seeing behavioral improvement, gratitude, or the sparks of a relationship.

"I have been benign and accepting with that kid for four months now, and he still hasn't changed. No matter how much you give him, he will never be satisfied. What he really needs is a good tough approach, not all of this attention. There are going to be some changes. . . ."

There is undoubtedly some realistic limit to the time any worker can be expected to spend in unfruitful efforts with a particular child without becoming discouraged. But the most effective worker will be the one who can maintain some optimism in the face of admittedly discouraging indications. Bettelheim, in a 1964 lecture at Wayne State University, suggested that it takes considerably longer to undo the problems of children than it originally took to create them. We cannot be certain that the day we abandoned our efforts would not have been the turning point; but we can be certain that when we give up on the child he himself will be moved one step closer to total futility.

Conclusion

In this chapter we have considered how the interactions of child-care workers with disturbed children are influenced by a great many factors beyond the official policies of the institution. The external pressures that must be dealt with by the worker as well as certain internal factors resulting from the worker's personality have been discussed under the general rubric of "needs of the child-care worker." The worker finds that he must, of necessity, conform at least minimally to institutional policy, satisfy his supervisors and superiors, be accepted by his co-workers, remain consistent with his philosophy and beliefs about human behavior, be able to control the children, achieve a modicum of success with a child, and finally be accepted by the children. In each instance, it has been demonstrated how these needs can conflict with the appropriate therapeutic handling of maladjusted children.

The foregoing should not imply that we feel all institutional procedures require radical alteration or that the personalities of workers need to be reconstructed; we are aware that it is notoriously difficult to change radically either social organizations or the people who staff them. What then would we recommend to alleviate these pressures and avoid these pitfalls? A beginning to the solution of any problem is becoming aware that there is a problem. Our first recommendation would be a careful assessment of the role of the child-care worker within the institution and a determination of how each worker views his role. We hope that our somewhat "universalized" list can function as a starting point of such an assessment. This is surely a more modest but more practical beginning than revolutionizing institutions or "therapizing" workers.

Much more effort must be made to involve higher level personnel in the real issues encountered by child-care workers in their everyday work. This does not imply that "meetings" between child-care workers and other personnel, if conducted in the traditional fashion, will do much good. Typically, such efforts at "communication" have resulted in either nondirective procedures where workers present their problems to a psychiatrist, psychologist, or social worker who makes minimal comments, or excessively directive methods where the clinical staff pass out interpretations and lecture to the child-care staff. The prevalence of both approaches is perhaps less related to their effectiveness than to the fact that the procedures avoid the conflict possible in a "give-and-take" interaction.

An atmosphere must be established where there is a real freedom for various staff members at all levels to communicate honestly about major issues (Matsushima, 1964). All too often an institution is full of people who are all trying to prove their infallibility to one another. If supervisory and clinical staff as well as child-care workers are free to acknowledge their own questions, doubts, and mistakes, it should be easier to focus upon the needs of children. It seems to us necessary that supervisory and clinical staff have regular opportunities to interact in the life of the cottage, perhaps substituting for child-care workers from time to time, eating with the youngsters occasionally, or joining the cottage group on special occasions. It seems very logical to involve only professionals with substantial line experience in the direct supervision of child-care workers.

The teaching of the technical skills of child-care work by personnel with "on-line" experience and perhaps current *in situ* involvement with the children is the most direct solution. The workers are most exposed to institutional pressures and pitfalls when they possess no real technical information about how to deal with the children. We must stop pretending that workers are "born" to the work. Even the search for research variables that assure success is a little pointless. We must work with the motivated individuals who come to our institutions' doors; let us begin by teaching them in groups and in individual supervision what we know about establishing relationships, about managing tantrums, activities, and routines. Such is the core knowledge about the management of children in groups that is directly relevant to child-care work. It is the technical detail of our trade. It does not "suffer in the translation" the way textbooks on child development or clinical studies of pathology do. Such topics may be useful as supplements, but they can no more tell us how to do our job than can the analysis of cement tell us how to construct a building.

In the last place, personal awareness is an important attribute of a successful child-care worker. Personal individual psychotherapy is certainly not the only means of expanding such awareness—and therapy for all is surely an impractical solution to training good child-care workers. The selection of child-care workers with some degree of self-awareness is a start, but, like many other aspects of professional roles, self-awareness can be taught in some degree. Sensitive supervision by line-experienced personnel who are familiar with the technical details of child-care work can and does help workers learn awareness. The more a worker knows of the details of the work—for example the management of an angry child—the better he can assess his behavior in the particular situation.

Child-care work can become a profession as it establishes a base of knowledge and skill; while some of this knowledge is borrowed from related professions, most must emanate from the practice of child care. We feel that the pressures and pitfalls common in child-care work can be best avoided as we teach the technical skills of child management. In addition, we see involving high-level personnel in everyday child-life issues, fostering an atmosphere of honest communication, and developing an awareness of our own behavior as essentials in quality child-care work. These are the foundations of the therapeutic milieu.

References

Bromberg, W. 1961. Symposium on psychopathy. *Archives of Criminal Psychodynamics,* Vol 4.

Carducci, Dewey J. 1962. A possible solution to the training and orienting of child-care workers. *Child Welfare,* 41(5): 212–216.

Grossbard, Hyman. 1960. *Cottage parents—what they have to be, know, and do.* New York: Child Welfare League of America.

Horney, Karen. 1937. *The neurotic personality of our time.* New York: W. W. Norton.

Matsushima, John. 1964. Communication and cottage parent supervision in a residential treatment center. *Child Welfare,* 43(10): 529–534.

Mayer, Morris F. 1958. *A guide for child-care workers.* New York: Child Welfare League of America.

———. 1963. Differentials in training child-care workers. In *Training of child-care staff.* New York: Child Welfare League of America.

POLSKY, HOWARD W. 1962. *Cottage Six—the social system of delinquent boys in residential treatment.* New York: Russell Sage Foundation.

REIK, THEODORE. 1963. *The need to be loved.* New York: Farrar, Strauss.

INDEX